Diabetes, Obesity, and Sexuality

Here are the latest facts and important information about:

DIABETES *and*

- obesity and sexuality • obesity and self-esteem
- child-bearing • cancer • hypoglycemia
- alcoholism • vegetarianism • nutrition
- altered sexual awareness • impotence
- hypertension • cardiovascular • estrogens

Including the most frequently asked QUESTIONS and ANSWERS about diabetes, CASE HISTORIES, MENU PLANS AND SUGGESTIONS, and a special chapter for Health Professionals.

About the authors

Sam Addanki, Ph.D., is an associate professor of pediatrics and assistant professor of physiological chemistry at the Ohio State University College of Medicine. He is a native of Madras, India, and holds degrees from the University of Madras, India, and from the Ohio State University. He is a member of the American Society of Biological Chemists, the American Diabetes Association, and the American Association of Cancer Research. He spent 1978 and 1979 at the Diabetes Research Center of the University of Pennsylvania Medical School, Philadelphia, completing research on diabetes.

Dr. Addanki has been a diabetic for the past 15 years and he controls the disease completely by a low-meat, low-fat, high fiber diet. He recently published the findings of his research in *Preventine Medicine*, an international journal. He is an ardent public speaker, and he is very active in public and community affairs.

Dr. Maria Simonson is Director of the Johns Hopkins Health Weight and Stress Clinic and holds an appointment as Assistant Professor in the Department of Psychiatry and Behavioral Sciences, School of Medicine.

Dr. S. V. Cherukuri is a medical staff member at Lorrain Community Hospital, Lorrain, Ohio.

DIABETES BREAKTHROUGH:
Control Through Nutrition

Sam Addanki, Ph.D.
Associate Professor, College of Medicine
The Ohio State University

with

Maria Simonson, Ph.D., Sc.D.
and
S.V. Cherukuri, M.D., F.R.C.S. (Edinburgh)

PINNACLE BOOKS   NEW YORK

This book is not intended to replace the services of a physician. Any application of the recommendations set forth in the following pages is at the reader's discretion and sole risk.

DIABETES BREAKTHROUGH:
CONTROL THROUGH NUTRITION

Copyright © 1982 by Somasundaram Addanki, Ph.D.

An original Pinnacle Books edition, published for the first time anywhere.

First printing, August 1982
Third printing, November 1983

ISBN: 0-523-41827-2

Printed in Canada

PINNACLE BOOKS, INC.
1430 Broadway
New York, New York 10018

The authors would like to thank the following for permission to quote passages and reprint tables and figures from other published works:

Academic Press, Inc.
Kawate, Ryoso, et al. 1978. Preliminary studies of the prevalence and mortality of diabetes mellitus an Japanese in Japan and on the island of Hawaii. In *Advances in Metabolic Disorders*, ed. by M. Miller and P.H. Bennett, vol. 9, p. 201.

Academic Press, Inc.
Addanki, Somasundaram. 1981. Roles of nutrition, obesity, estrogens in diabetes mellitus. *Preventive Medicine*, vol. 10, no. 5.

Fredericks, Carlton
Breast Cancer, originally published by Grosset and Dunlap Publishers, Inc., 1977, p. 169.

Grune & Stratton, Inc.
Cohen, A.M. 1961. Prevalence of diabetes among different ethnic Jewish groups in Israel. *Metabolism* 10:50.

The Lancet
Singh, Inder. 1955. Low fat diet and therapeutic doses of insulin in diabetes mellitus. *The Lancet*, 26 Feb. issue.

Metropolitan Life Insurance Company
How you can control your weight, p. 2. Tables based

on data from the *Build and Blood Pressure Study*, 1959, published by the Society of Actuaries.

New England Journal of Medicine
Harwood, Reed. 1957. Severe diabetes with remission: Report of a case and review of the literature. *New England Journal of Medicine* 257:257-61.

Royal Society of Medicine
Himsworth, H.P. 1949. Diet in the aetiology of human diabetes. *Proceedings of the Royal Society of Medicine* 42:323-26.

Stein and Day Publishers
1974. *Psychodietetics*, © 1974 by E. Cheraskin, M.D., D.M.D. and William M. Ringsdorf, Jr., D.M.D., M.S. with Arline Brecher. Quote from Dr. Joseph Wilder, p. 77.

**DEDICATED
to the
SERVICE
of
MANKIND**

Acknowledgments

Writing, like research, is often a lonely job. Without the company of a stimulating team of family, friends, and colleagues, I would have found it intolerable. In this spirit I sincerely thank the following persons.

All readers of the book are actually enjoying a "translation" by Bob and Patricia Hill, two Americans who offered their services to substitute readable layman's English for my scientific jargon. Russ Walker, Corinne Smith, and Dr. Samuel Meites provided valuable suggestions to smooth out my occasional slips of the pen. Immaculate final typing was done by Dorothea Rienstra.

Any researcher owes a tremendous debt to all previous work in his field. I would like especially to thank Dr. Meites, Dr. Bandaru Reddy, Dr. R. V. Panganamala, Dr. Harold Wilson, Dr. Dhananjaya Kamisette, Dr. M.S.N. Murthy, Dr. C. M. Thorne, Professor Arthur Cullman, and Professor K. N. Rao for advice and critique, without which any scientific effort is only unchallenged opinion.

I would also like to thank Don Gorman, Millie Rinehart, and Jerry Harvey for their help in marketing, art work, and medical photography respectively.

Professional advice in nonmedical areas was provided by attorney Jerry Simon Chasen and financial consultants Jon McGinty, Bob Wills, and Bill Brame.

I owe a word of thanks for the stimulating environments provided by the Ohio State University, the University of Pennsylvania, and the Children's Hospital Research Foundation.

I would also like to thank Charles Woods and June Lazerus of Pinnacle Books, for a job well done.

Finally, proving that the support of wife and family is a necessary part of any successful venture, I would like to thank my wife, Sathya, for standing by me, literally through "thick and thin," sickness and health, and every other adverse condition imaginable. At times she was the only positive factor, and no other author can more truthfully say, "Without her this book would not have been possible."

SAM ADDANKI, Ph.D.
Associate Professor, College of Medicine,
Ohio State University
Children's Hospital, Columbus, Ohio

Contents

Foreword

Diabetes Breakthrough: Control Through Nutrition, is an interesting and timely book. It is an important and welcome contribution to the expanding effort to alert the general public to the increasing dangers created by the major chronic degenerative diseases, of which diabetes is one.

Dr. Sam Addanki and his contributing authors, Dr. Maria Simonson and Dr. S. V. Cherukuri, are to be congratulated for their very valuable contributions toward our increased knowledge of the causes of diabetes, as well as its prevention and treatment.

Especially noteworthy is the splendid documentation of medical facts well known to those of us who are constantly seeing patients stricken by preventable and postponable sicknesses. The frank discussion of the sexual problems of obese and diabetic people is to be commended.

Enough medical research data are presented in this book to make it very evident that malnutrition and malabsorption stalk the people of our land. Obesity, it is made quite clear, does not indicate a well-nourished individual; on the contrary, it creates a chain reaction of nonhealthful body conditions.

There are always different viewpoints in medicine as to the relative importance of various causative factors. There is no doubt in my mind, however, that the authors' analysis of the causes and prevention of diabetes and obesity is quite logical, and Dr. Addanki receives my wholehearted support and concurrence.

Dr. John Knowles, former president of the Rockefeller Foundation, has stated, "The next major advance in the health of the American people will result only from what the individual is willing to do for himself." The harm that has been done by the effects of our Westernized diets and the overwhelmingly anti-nutrition environment created by our poisoned, polluted world, as pointed out in my book *"Coronary? Cancer? God's Answer?,* is emphasized in this work. It gives new hope to the American people, who can increase their chances for better health and a longer, more productive life through improved diet, food supplements, and a positive attitude.

Diabetes Breakthrough: Control Through Nutrition is a dynamic, well-documented analysis of the major causes of this chronic degenerative disease and includes simple, clear-out preventive measures. Dr. Addanki alerts his readers to the mass of misinformation that imprisons our minds and misleads many Americans to a mediocre, unhappy, unhealthy, and substandard existence.

If this book succeeds in reaching these unfortunate people and brings to light the fact that they can lead happy, normal, sexually fulfilled lives, then it will have served its purpose well.

Proverbs 17:22 admonishes us: "A joyful heart is the health of the body, but a depressed spirit dries up the bones." Good nutrition lies at the root of much joy.

R. O. BRENNAN, D.O., M.D., PH.G., D.P.H., F.A.P.M., F.I.C.A.N., F.A.C.G.P. AUTHOR OF NUTRIGENETICS AND CORONARY? CANCER? GOD'S ANSWER: PREVENT IT! MEDICAL DIRECTOR, BRENNAN PREVENTIVE MEDICINE CENTER AND SOUTHWEST FOUNDATION OF PREVENTIVE MEDICINE

Preface

There are many good books, both old and new, on the subject of diabetes mellitus. Generally, they describe the disease, and then go on to tell you how to adjust your life to the regimen of insulin use, exchange diets, exercise, and blood and urine measurement. The picture they paint is one of resignation and plodding courage.

But how many of you know, for instance, that juvenile-onset diabetes and adult-onset diabetes are two *completely* different disorders? What if I told you that the disease the other books talk about affects only 5 percent of all diabetics? What if I told you that 90 percent of recently diagnosed diabetics can *totally reverse* their condition? What if I told you that 75 percent of all obese persons eventually become diabetic? What if I told you that many insulin-dependent diabetics can discontinue the drug? In this book, I am going to prove each fact to you, step by step.

The first thing you may want to ask is, "Who is Sam Addanki? Why should I trust him?" I will tell you my story, both personal and professional. You will learn what events led me to spend over sixteen years searching for the cause of diabetes. When you finish the book, you should know the latest facts about this little-understood disease.

In talking to other diabetics, I have found that the most common area of confusion is the difference between juvenile-onset and adult-onset diabetes. Juvenile diabetes strikes youngsters between the ages of two and fourteen. For one reason or another, the pancreas stops producing insulin. These are the diabetics that will need insulin for the rest of their lives. For them there are many good books about their disorder and how to cope with it. Fortunately, only between 5 and 10 percent of diabetics are this type.

The majority of diabetics, and virtually all of those diagnosed after the age of twenty-five, have adult-onset diabetes. This disorder is *not hereditary*. It is degenerative. I will prove to you that heredity accounts for only 8 percent of diabetes, while poor eating habits account for over 90 percent.

One way of determining whether a disease is hereditary or not is to compare the incidence and prevalence of the disease in different countries. Then, by noticing what happens when members of one society move to another area, we can see the effects of the new environment. We shall investigate what happened when various groups of Jews migrated to Israel. We shall explore the influences of diet, heredity, and environment on Japanese migrating to Hawaii, and on three groups of Eastern Indians—those migrating to Natal, South Africa; those who went to Trinidad, West Indies; and those who moved to Fiji. These studies and others throughout the book reveal some amazing facts about the cause of diabetes.

Continuing the search for the cause of this disease, I noticed that more women get diabetes than men. This led me to the study of various factors that could cause women to be more prone to the disease. Along with the statistics concerning the rates of diabetes in women around the world, we will consider the effects of childbearing, birth-control pills, hormone treatments, and diet on susceptibility to diabetes.

Of course, men get diabetes too. But men in Western countries get it much more often than men in Asian or African countries. It is necessary to look into the differences in lifestyle between Asian and Western countries to determine the reasons why American men have more problems with the disease. It turns out that men in Western countries such as the United States, have fallen into certain habits that directly affect the degree to which they are susceptible to degenerative diseases.

Obesity is one of these factors. It is related to all types of degenerative diseases and to certain other problems that have not been understood until now. In both men and women, obesity is one of the main causes not only of diabetes but of a whole list of complaints, both physical and mental. You will find out how to avoid or even *reverse* the effects of obesity and banish the related complaints forever.

Since the human body is really just one big chemical factory, it should not come as a surprise that what affects one part of the body can affect another part as well. Such is the case with the reproductive system, which is one part of the whole and yet is not immune from the deficiencies of the rest of the body. Problems of impotency, libido, and sexuality in general can often be traced to the physical changes brought about by poor nutrition. I will explain this aspect fully and offer suggestions to the sufferers.

Normal growth of the cells can take place only when proper nutrition is available. It makes sense, then, that abnormal growth of the cells may be related to abnormal nutrition. With this in mind, we will look at how diet is related to four types of cancer, and the implications for preventing these killers. The relationship between obesity and cancer will also be discussed.

Almost everyone has experienced low blood sugar. There is a disorder called *hypoglycemia* which is related to diabetes and which causes the sufferer to experience this feeling daily. In my research concerning diabetes, I learned a lot about hypoglycemia, and I will pass this information along to you.

Another nutritional problem, common in the United States and elsewhere, is alcohol abuse. We will consider it here, because it has a direct effect on degenerative diseases in general, and on diabetes in particular.

I don't want to give you all these facts about diabetes

without giving some suggestions about prevention and treatment as well. I feel that by following the guidelines in the latter chapters of this book you will be able to avoid or reverse many conditions you and others may have considered inevitable or attributable to "old age." Even the widely publicized loss of sex drive in men can in many cases be reversed through nutritional therapy. It has been proved that this phenomenon is not due to any natural aging process.

Because many of the nutrients and vitamins normally present in food are removed or destroyed between the time the food is harvested and the time you eat it, a section on supplements is provided. I have attempted to walk a middle path between the "minimum daily requirement" recommended by the U.S. government and the "megadose" amounts suggested by some popular books. The minimum amounts will keep an average-sized person from getting scurvy or pellagra, but I do not believe that this is total health. On the other hand, amounts approaching ten thousand times the minimum daily allowance may be wasteful. My recommendations are intended to keep you totally fit and healthy, but are conservative enough to keep you from passing the most expensive urine on your block.

I have included a chapter of questions and answers taken from my lectures and seminars, taking great care to choose the most frequently asked questions as well as those with a broad range of application. For best results, please read the entire chapter.

One exciting, relatively new subject that is always popular at seminars is vegetarianism. I include a chapter on this development because of the variety of diets and diet groups which have sprung up in recent years.

Samples of menus for both weight loss and weight maintenance are included. From these, the reader can create new meal plans that not only will be nutritious but will enable him to avoid obesity and diabetes, two of the most serious problems facing affluent Western societies.

In any discussion of how foods affect the body, certain technical words are unavoidable. In the interest of clarity, a complete glossary is included to assist the reader's understanding of the material.

As you go from chapter to chapter, some of the ideas will seem familiar. I certainly did not discover them all. For the last twelve years, research the world over has hinted at the problems of modern nutrition. After reading *why* this type of eating causes so many degenerative diseases, you will not only know what to do, you will do it—because no rational person would slowly kill himself on purpose. I was diabetic for many years before I discovered why. Don't hesitate! There are two types of people—those who learn and grow, and the other kind. Turn the page and TAKE CHARGE OF YOUR SYMPTOMS AND YOUR LIFE!

SAM ADDANKI, Ph.D.
Columbus, Ohio

1

Sam

In India

I was born on March 7, 1932, into a family of ten children—seven girls and three boys. Two brothers died from accidents as youngsters.

My family was financially comfortable and provided me with a good education and a healthy environment in which to grow. My father, however, became increasingly obese and was eventually diagnosed as a diabetic. I became curious about this disease and often wondered what caused it and why it seemed to affect his personality and even his normal sexual awareness.

I continued my education in India by completing a two-year college in 1951 and a five-year B.Sc. program in 1957. In 1954 I got married and started a family. I was healthy and lean, and my wife and I enjoyed a normal, fulfilling married life. I worked in India for three years for the government of Andhra Pradesh. My father became progressively worse. With each increase in his suffering, my interest in diabetes sharpened. In 1960 I came alone to the United States to continue my education and pursue what had become an all-consuming obsession.

In America

I weighed a lean 125 pounds (on a 5'6½" frame) when I arrived, and lived with an American family for one

1

year. They introduced me to the typical American food habits, which would haunt me for years to come. Bacon and sausage for breakfast, and heaps of jelly on white bread! Dinners with meatballs, steak, pork, and other Western treats! I strayed from the semi-vegetarian, whole-wheat ways of my early married years in India. Of course I gained weight, but the thought of it being a problem never occurred to me. "How could anyone get diabetes in the U.S.A.?" I asked. "It's so hygienic here." I had no inkling that obesity and diabetes were related. My blood pressure rose, but I attributed it to long hours of hard work.

In 1961, I moved out of my "foster" home and lived alone. I had learned to cook American dishes, but I had not learned how to prepare individual portions. Hour after hour of education was accompanied by pound after pound of food. On occasion I could devour whole trays of meatballs, packages of bacon, and quarts of soda pop. Gradually I became obese, weighing 185 pounds, with blood pressure to match. Meanwhile, I obtained a Master of Science degree in 1962, and a Ph.D. in 1964 in physiology, biochemistry, nutrition, and endocrinology.

My wife, Sathya, and our two daughters came over from India in 1964. Sathya had been a vegetarian in our native land, but once in the United States she adopted Westernized eating habits. As you will see later, her behavior is common to all migrating people, and it tipped me off to an important fact about diabetes. From a svelte 94 pounds on a 5'4" frame, she ballooned to 160 pounds. She also started taking birth-control pills, and they seemed to make her grow more affectionate as the months passed. Sexual activity was becoming her primary concern, and frankly I was puzzled, even a bit scared, because I was unable to accommodate her increasing needs.

In 1966, with all of the "classic" symptoms—thirst, polyuria, pains, and dizziness—I went to the doctor and was diagnosed a diabetic. He put me on a 1000-calorie-per-day, "exchange-type" diet.

2

A normal healthy man, after separation from his wife for four years, would be something of a sexpot upon her arrival. But for some unexplained reason, our sexual relations were few, and my own interest was low. And this condition lasted for years! At one point I was actually impotent, and my wife, assuming that this was a permanent condition, threatened divorce. At that time of my life, naturally, my mental state reached rock bottom.

In 1974, to improve my health, I began a program of jogging. Every morning I would get up early and exercise for thirty minutes. Then I would jog for fifteen to thirty minutes and then exercise again. This provided me with more physical vigor, but I was still not satisfied with my progress.

In 1976 I took some training in Transcendental Meditation (TM) and practiced it daily for two years. In India I had been exposed to TM but did not learn it. Ironically, I had to pay someone in Columbus, Ohio, a stiff fee to teach it to me. While it gave a boost to my daily work, it did not help my "family problem" any. To a small degree it helped my blood pressure. Meanwhile, that year, my wife was also diagnosed as diabetic.

During my sabbatical year of research at the University of Pennsylvania, in 1978, I tried to follow a regimen of long work hours. We lived about fifteen miles from the old building where I worked. I had to get up at 4 A.M., jog, meditate, dress, eat, and then embark on a one-hour journey on wheels and foot to reach the campus. When I arrived I climbed five flights of stairs to reach my office. By 8 A.M. I was so exhausted that I could not adequately do the work I so desperately wanted to do.

In a search for help on my problem I came upon a cassette program by Dennis Waitley which suggested "biofeedback" as a method of controlling one's energy. I enrolled in a fourteen-week course at nearby Thomas Jefferson Medical School, again parting with a stiff fee. We were strapped for money because of the one-third cut in pay I had taken to enjoy the sabbatical leave, but I was determined to make the most of it.

Biofeedback turned out to be a thousand times better than TM for increasing my stamina. I included it in my morning routine, along with music to stimulate my mind. My work day was now charged with energy and often would last until 7 or 8 P.M., with no problems of fatigue or lack of concentration. At dinner time I would "recharge" with biofeedback, music, and food, and I could continue effectively for several more hours. I felt as though I were getting thirty-six hours of work done in twenty-four hours. Rather than meditating transcendentally, I would spend one hour each day just "plain thinking."

It seemed that I had conquered every problem I had—except one. My sex life was still poor, my marriage still threatened. Because my interest had increased somewhat, I wondered what had caused it. While working on the cause of diabetes, I studied the pancreas of the freshwater carp. Unknowingly, I had part of the answer right under my nose.

We used so many carp in the laboratory that my colleagues and I thought about selling the unused portions for extra money. Fortunately for me, the university would not allow it, so we split the fish up and took them home for food. The fish in my diet now displaced much of the dietary fat of my "meatball" days.

Suddenly, in April 1979, the pieces of my theory fell into place. As you read each chapter, I will explain how this insight developed. I learned finally what I believe causes diabetes, and, as a bonus, I realized how to save my marriage. By July 1979, I had totally controlled both my wife's and my own diabetes, and our marriage, instead of being like a brother-sister relationship, resembled that of a couple of giggling newlyweds.

So there you have it—a brief history of me, my family, and my research. It is not the details of the search that should concern you, however, but the results. To this day, because of my high-fiber, low-fat diet, I have no diabetic symptoms and no sexual dysfunction. You

4

too can enjoy this freedom, by learning how to take charge of your symptoms and beat diabetes through diet.

LET'S GET STARTED!

2

Diabetes Connection

Scientific theories can't be proved by personal stories or unique observations. For that reason, large groups of subjects must be observed in a very careful way. Feeling that the complications of maturity-onset diabetes can be controlled by diet, I set out to determine the relative importance of heredity, environment, and diet as causes of this disease. In this chapter, I shall briefly discuss diabetes itself and then show you how I isolated diet as the main causative factor. I will limit this chapter to maturity-onset diabetes (diabetes mellitus), which generally strikes adult men and women between the ages of forty and sixty. And I will show that often the crippling symptoms can be avoided.

For too long you have heard that if one or both of your parents had diabetes, you are 100 percent doomed to suffer from it sooner or later. One person I know adopted an attitude of "If I'm going to die early anyway, I might as well live it up while I still can." This man eats, drinks, and smokes with no regard for tomorrow, let alone for his later years. Courting danger seems to be a socially accepted national pastime, especially among men. This new evidence should shock my friend, and others like him, into realizing that we determine our own future suffering, in this case, by over 90 percent.

A diabetic's system can't use insulin effectively. He often has plenty, but its inefficient use leads to roller-coaster swings in his blood-sugar level. These, in turn, lead to a nightmare of painful and embarrassing symptoms. As the blood sugar level rises and isn't used, two things happen: (1) sugar spills into the urine, and (2) the liver starts busily creating glucose out of fat and protein. You don't want the latter to happen because the protein comes from your muscles, and the fat causes multiple problems in your system. Fat-related ketones are dumped into your bloodstream; their acidity causes dehydration, nausea, and labored breathing, then coma and death.

Others have suspected that heredity and environment weren't the only factors causing this disease. Our contribution is in demonstrating not only that diet *is* a factor but that (1) it is the most important one, and (2) it can be controlled by the victim.

Diabetes is no small problem, and it is getting worse. In 1975, the National Commission of Diabetes reported that there were 10 million diabetics in the United States. By 1980, the number had grown to 15 million, a 50 percent increase in just 5 years.

It came to my attention that there was a tremendous difference in the number of deaths due to diabetes among different countries (Figure 2.1). I found a significantly higher proportion of deaths among females— twice as many or more in many countries. In Luxembourg, the death rate from diabetes was more than two and a half times higher in women. In Finland, it was twice as high. In the United States the female/male ratio was 1.39. That means for every 100 men who died from diabetes in this country, 139 women died from it. More recently, researchers have found, by studying examples of countries with similar stress levels, cultural norms and behavior patterns, that the influence of these factors is minimal. Measurement of the incidence of diabetes in migrating peoples suggested various before-and-after studies. Previous studies by Albert Damon had shown that race was not important in genetic diseases. Also, genetic changes don't occur over the short run. Therefore, we can get legitimate evidence on dietary factors by studying migrating people over a five-to

7

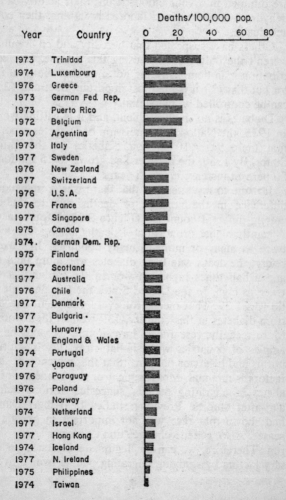

Figure 2.1

AGE-ADJUSTED DEATH RATES
FOR DIABETES MELLITUS

MALE

Deaths/100,000 pop.

Year	Country
1973	Trinidad
1974	Luxembourg
1976	Greece
1973	German Fed. Rep.
1973	Puerto Rico
1972	Belgium
1970	Argentina
1973	Italy
1977	Sweden
1976	New Zealand
1977	Switzerland
1976	U.S.A.
1976	France
1977	Singapore
1975	Canada
1974	German Dem. Rep.
1975	Finland
1977	Scotland
1977	Australia
1976	Chile
1977	Denmark
1977	Bulgaria
1977	Hungary
1977	England & Wales
1974	Portugal
1977	Japan
1976	Paraguay
1976	Poland
1977	Norway
1974	Netherland
1977	Israel
1977	Hong Kong
1974	Iceland
1977	N. Ireland
1975	Philippines
1974	Taiwan

Figure 2.1
AGE-ADJUSTED DEATH RATES
FOR DIABETES MELLITUS

FEMALE

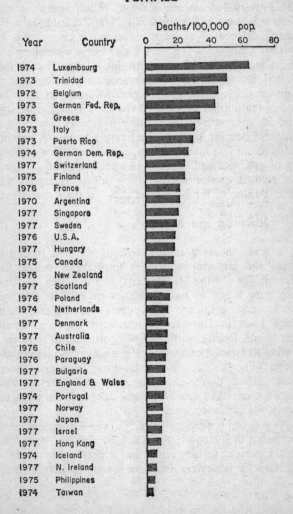

twenty-year period, as they adopt the eating habits of their new neighbors.

When in Rome . . .

The groups studied were as follows: (1) Jews migrating to Israel, (2) Japanese migrating to Hawaii, and (3) Eastern Indians migrating to Natal, South Africa; Trinidad, West Indies; and Fiji, New Zealand. In each case, incidence of diabetes increased after moving. If you are tempted to say, "So what, I'm not planning on migrating anywhere," consider this. If you live in the United States, or any other place that encourages a high-fat, high-sugar, low-fiber diet, then you may be one of ten million "cooking diabetics." That is a person who is unknowingly incubating a future case of the "sugars" because of ill-advised eating habits. A person tends to eat like his neighbors, because of the availability of products and because of social pressures. When the studied groups moved, they politely adopted the killer cuisine of the host countries—to their detriment.

Jews on the Move

In a study of more than ten thousand men from six areas, the importance of diet to diabetes started to emerge. Jews in the Middle East, North Africa, and Israel were found to have a higher prevalence (known cases) and incidence (new cases) of diabetes than those born in Europe. Comparisons between immigrants and locally born groups showed that Jews migrating to Israel increased their chances of becoming diabetic (Figure 2.2), European-born Jews and those from Africa don't generally contract diabetes, but among those that moved to and adopted the ways of Israel, the incidence rose.

As you can see from Figure 2.2., the old settlers have succeeded in increasing their rate of diabetes from less than 1 percent to between 6 and 8 percent, by accepting Israel's lifestyles. Put more simply, before they

10

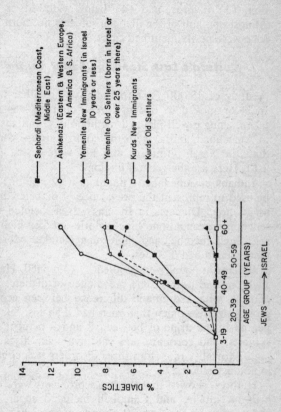

Figure 2.2

JEWISH ETHNIC DISTRIBUTION
PREVALENCE OF DIABETICS IN ISRAEL

- ■ Sephardi (Mediterranean Coast, Middle East)
- ○ Ashkenazi (Eastern & Western Europe, N. America & S. Africa)
- ▲ Yemenite New Immigrants (in Israel 10 years or less)
- △ Yemenite Old Settlers (born in Israel or over 25 years there)
- □ Kurds New Immigrants
- ● Kurds Old Settlers

% DIABETICS

14
12
10
8
6
4
2
0

AGE GROUP (YEARS)

3-19   20-39   40-49   50-59   60+

JEWS ——→ ISRAEL

moved, only 1 person out of 100 or more had diabetes. After living in Israel for 5 or 10 years, 6 to 8 persons per 100 were affected. These travelers simply ate themselves to bad health. Other factors associated with diabetes among Jews were: (1) overweight, (2) low education, (3) divorce, and (4) being widowed or single. Almost one-half of the diabetic subjects not born in Europe were newly identified cases.

Custard's Last Stand, or Sugar vs. Indians

A study of 45,000 Eastern Indians who either lived in India or moved to one of three countries was undertaken, using a well-planned methodology. Indians living in Amedabad, India, were the control group, while Indians in Natal, Trinidad, and Fiji were tested (Table 2.1). Here are the general findings:

Indians in Amedabad (population: 2 million) could be used to represent the prevalence of diabetes in India as a whole. Diabetes in Indians was associated with a sedentary occupation, high calorie intake, high birth rate, high income, and high sugar intake. More men than women had diabetes.

Indians in Natal were studied by Campbell, Hathorn, Jackson, and others. The prevalence of diabetes was 6 percent, with a dramatic difference between economic groups. More women than men had diabetes. Sugar appeared in the urine of between 8 and 9 percent of the subjects, and coronary and cardiovascular disease was high. Mortality rate from these disorders was confirmed in autopsy studies.

Hathorn showed that the heart problems were due to high fat intake, and Campbell included sugar intake and obesity (more than 20 pounds overweight) as culprits. Jackson, however, pointed out that genetic differences were unavoidable in the studies.

Over 9,000 Indians in Trinidad were studied, starting in 1961; at that time, Indians were one-third of the population. The affluence factor showed up here, as did male predominance. Other factors noticed were:

12

Table 2.1
Summary of Investigations on Indians in India, Indians in Natal, Indians in Trinidad and Indians in Fiji

Indians in	Age group	Population	Sample Studied	Sex Ratio F/M	% Known Cases	% Newly Discovered	Total Rate %	Keto-Acidosis	Juvenile Diabetes	Obesity—% of Diabetes	Year Studied	Years Migrated
Ahmedabad (India)	>15	1 million	6987	0.51	1.65	1.39	3.04	rare	rare	16	1975	—
Natal (South Africa)	>10	60,000 in 1963	2427	1.45	1.8	4.2	6.0	rare	rare	17.8	1968	100
Trinidad (West Indies)	all ages	302,100 in 1960	9421	0.91	1.13	2.32	3.45	rare	rare	39	1961	50
Fiji (New Zealand)	>21	208,943 in 1966	1000	0.68	3.8	1.9	5.7	rare	rare	49	1964–1965	100

(1) an increase in diabetes with advancing age; (2) obesity in 40 percent of the diabetics; (3) twice as many new cases as known ones; (4) few juvenile cases; (5) low fat intake; (6) high sugar intake; (7) higher frequency in females with more than five children; and (8) an association of multiparity (bearing more than one child), overweight, and diabetes.

Out of 1,000 Indians studied in Fiji, men were again the losers in the fight against diabetes. Of the Indians in Fiji, 5.7 percent were diagnosed diabetic, and almost one-half (mostly women) were overweight. Over 90 percent of the diabetics had coronary heart disease. Cassidy found that the only environmental factors involved here were food availability and obesity.

In conclusion, the Indian studies have shown that several factors are almost always implicated. Obesity was always a factor, especially in Trinidad, where the consumption of rum is high among males. Being in the 50-percent tax bracket didn't help, either. Invariably, more affluent Indians had diabetes than their less fortunate counterparts. In India, 18 percent of affluent Indians had diabetes, while only 2 percent of poorer ones did. A Westernized diet is nutritional Russian roulette, pure and simple. Obesity and a high-fat-sugar diet are clearly the enemies, especially during the danger years between thirty and forty.

Hawaii—Land of Opportunity

We all *know* that the "poor" Japanese eat rice at every meal, with maybe a few undercooked vegetables. Let's bring them to the United States and put a little "meat on their bones." If we did, we'd be doing them a great disservice, because when Japanese migrate to Hawaii and eat a Westernized diet, diabetes increases almost threefold.

When Japanese in Japan and Hawaii were compared, other variables besides diet were carefully controlled. In Hawaii various groups live and work in a similar climate and under comparable physiological conditions.

These investigations were conducted by Kawate. As subjects, matching pairs (27) of relatives were selected for similar age, sex, and physical activities. There were 429 subjects in Hawaii; 182 between 40 and 59 and 247 over 60. The prevalence of diabetes in the Hawaiian group was between 1.5 and 2.6 times that in the Japanese sample. In fact, the prevalence of hyperlipemia, hypertriglyceridemia, and cardiac disease was higher in the Hawaiian group.

What was different? You're getting the picture, aren't you? Increased fat was again the culprit. Cholesterol in the blood is one way of measuring dietary fat. Japanese women in Hawaii had *triple* the blood cholesterol of the Hiroshima-based group.

Table 2.2

COMPARISON OF CALORIC INTAKE AND SPECIFIC NUTRIENTS

Nutrient	Japan (45–69 yrs.)	Hawaii (45–69 yrs.)
	% Intake	
protein	14.3	16.7
fat	15.1	33.2
alcohol	8.7	3.7
total calories	2132	2274

Bombs Away!

I wouldn't start a war to improve health, but Dr. Percy Stocks graphically showed that diabetes in England plummeted during both world wars. That sounds insane until we realize that wartime food rationing usually lowers our intake of fats and sweets. When fatty beef and

15

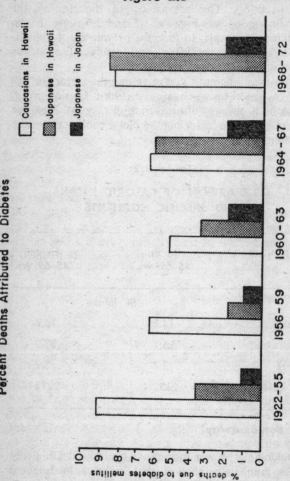

Figure 2.3

Percent Deaths Attributed to Diabetes

Legend:
- □ Caucasians in Hawaii
- ▨ Japanese in Hawaii
- ■ Japanese in Japan

Y-axis: % deaths due to diabetes mellitus (0–10)

X-axis: 1922-55, 1956-59, 1960-63, 1964-67, 1968-72

(Kawate, R. et al: Adv. Metab. Disorders 9: 201, 1978)

16

pork are reduced, along with ice cream and pastries, the body benefits. Sounds like Someone meant it that way!

Speaking of Sweets

When the presence of sugar was studied along with fat content in the diets of twenty-two countries, death rate was also shown to be affected. Persons eating a Western-type diet are between five and ten times as likely to get diabetes as those restricting their fat and sugar intake. The consumption of fats and sugar has increased dramatically, while complex carbohydrate intake is down. The last category (which includes vegetables, fruits, and grains) provides bulk, decreases intestinal bacterial activity, and helps prevent diabetes, obesity, and colon cancer.

In order for our habits to change, we will have to spend more time exploring the food we buy and the consequences of eating it. The basic requirements of life are food, shelter, and clothing. How many of us spend the same amount of time choosing meals as we do selecting a home or a suit of clothes? And yet neither of those affects us nearly as much.

1976 Diabetic Olympics

In comparing the United States to two other world societies, a final dramatic case can be made (Figure 2.5). In African society, 0.4 percent of the population has diabetes. That translates to 400 cases of diabetes for every 100,000 people. In Japan, the number is less than 500. But in America, at least 5 percent (5,000 per 100,000 people) have diabetes. And remember, these are only *diagnosed* diabetics. It doesn't even include borderline diabetics and those people who are sure to develop the disease unless they change their eating habits. Fat and sugar eaters become obese. And three out of every four obese people eventually get diabetes.

Using the techniques of cancer research, I have determined that the causative factors for diabetes in this

17

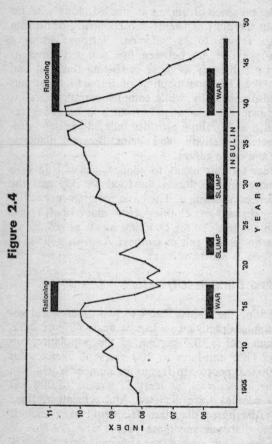

Figure 2.4

FIG. 1.—England and Wales. Diabetic mortality: comparative mortality indices (1938 basis). Showing the effect of food restrictions on diabetic mortality. (The figures for 1946 and 1947 have kindly been supplied by Dr. Percy Stocks.)

Courtesy of the Royal Society of Medicine

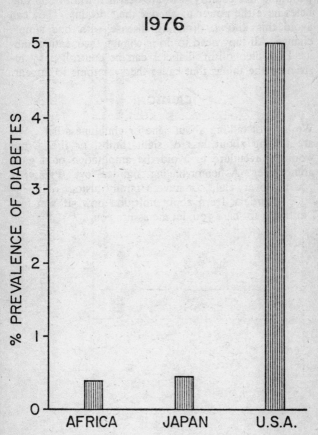

Figure 2.5

1976

% PREVALENCE OF DIABETES

AFRICA   JAPAN   U.S.A.

country are: 8 percent heredity, 0.6 percent environment, and 91.4 percent diet. This finding sheds new light on the current belief that heredity is the major factor. What it means, in effect, is that 9 out of every 10 people in this country who are destined to develop diabetes have the power to change their destiny. They can avoid this killing, disabling disease with one simple change. All they need to do is change their eating habits. Like alcoholism, diabetes can be controlled by restricting the things that cause the symptoms to appear.

CAUTION!

We are not talking about acne or chubbiness here. We are talking about loss of sight, limbs, or life. What would you endure to avoid the amputation of a gangrenous leg? A hemorrhaging, sightless eye? Please, if you are overweight, or have a family history of metabolic disorders, learn about nutrition now! If you feel I'm trying to scare you, let me assure you, I AM!

3

Women, Parity, and Diabetes

Women, we men are genuinely sorry. Through our actions, we have forced you to carry on a lifelong affair with a seductive but dangerous partner. You become acquainted with this fickle friend during puberty, continue the relationship in your childbearing years, intensify the encounters as your children grow, and cling to the rewards and memories in your middle and later life. The changeable chum to which I refer is the hormone estrogen, and the effects of this chemical on your body are what this chapter is about. Some of the actions of estrogen are perfectly normal, but, as with any good thing, more is not always better. The reason I feel that men should take some of the blame for the excess use of estrogen is that often such use is for cosmetic rather than valid medical reasons. When a doctor prescribes any medication, the known hazards must be weighed against the benefits.

In puberty, estrogens produced in the body help set in motion the process by which the little girl becomes a young woman. This phenomenon is not only normal but highly desirable. Later, during pregnancy, estrogens in the body increase and promote all the necessary requirements for the development of a healthy baby. Many women, when their families are big enough, use birth-control pills to prevent future pregnancies. Finally, during change of life, estrogens are often taken for various reasons. I will present some statistics on the health problems of women, and then show how some of these might be related to estrogen use.

After many years of research, I have noticed a clear pattern regarding the health of women compared to men. In this discussion, it is helpful to divide women into two age groups: seventeen to forty-four, and forty-five and over. These categories represent (roughly) the child-bearing years and the post-menopausal years. Also, I will first discuss the statistics for the United States, after which I will consider the diabetes figures for the rest of the world.

In 1973, the most recent year for which information is available, American women in both age groups had more prevalence *and* incidence of diabetes than men (Tables 3.1 + 3.2). As you can see, for every 1,000

Table 3.1

PREVALENCE OF DIABETES
in U.S.A. for 1973

Rate/1,000 pop.

	AGE (yrs)	
	17–44	45 and over
Male	6.9	48.12
Female	10.8	68.86

—Diabetes Data 1977 (USPHS)

Table 3.2

ANNUAL INCIDENCE OF DIABETES
in U.S.A. for 1973

Rate/1,000 pop.

	AGE (yrs)	
	17–44	45 and over
Male	1.5	5.5
Female	2.8	8.7

—Diabetes Data 1977 (USPHS)

persons, female prevalence was 10.8 and 68.86 for the two age groups! Men's rates were only 6.9 and 48.12. Incidence for women was 2.8 and 8.7, while for men it was only 1.5 and 5.5 per 1,000. In addition, more women than men die from diabetes each year (see Figure 2.1). Until now there has been no positive reason given for this discrepancy.

The problem is bad and getting worse. Between 1966 and 1973, the prevalence of diabetes in the United States increased by 41 percent (Table 3.3). Among

Table 3.3

CHANGES IN PREVALENCE OF REPORTED DIABETES BETWEEN 1965/66 AND 1973 HEALTH INTERVIEW SURVEY—UNITED STATES

	Rates per 1,000 persons 1965/66	1973	Percentage Change
All Persons	14.5	20.4	+41%
Males			
All Ages	12.9	16.3	+26%
<45	3.7	4.3	+16%
45–64	29.6	40.6	+37%
65+	51.4	60.3	+17%
Females			
All Ages	16.1	24.1	+50%
<45	3.8	6.8	+79%
45–64	31.0	44.4	+43%
65+	70.5	91.3	+29%

Source: Health Interview Survey 1965/66 and 1973, National Center for Health Statistics.

men, the increase was between 17 percent and 37 percent. The women, however, increased their prevalence more dramatically. Overall, their increase was 50 percent, but those under 45 posted a whopping 79 percent change between 1966 and 1973!

There are racial differences in the prevalence of diabetes (Table 3.4). Whites in the age groups under 45

Table 3.4

CHANGES IN PREVALENCE OF REPORTED DIABETES BETWEEN 1964/65 AND 1973 HEALTH INTERVIEW SURVEY—UNITED STATES

	Rates per 1,000 persons 1964/65	1973	Percentage Change
White			
All Ages	12.1	19.9	+64%
<45	3.0	5.3	+77%
45+	32.8	51.4	+57%
Non-white			
All Ages	13.3	23.9	+80%
<45	2.8	7.0	+150%
45+	50.2	80.3	+60%

Source: Health Interview Survey 1964/65 and 1973, National Center for Health Statistics.

and over 45 increased their prevalence 77 percent and 57 percent. Nonwhites in the same age groups posted increases of 150 percent and 60 percent! It is interesting to note how diabetes correlates with obesity (Table 3.5). As the table shows, the percentage of females

Table 3.5

**PERCENT OF OBESE INDIVIDUALS IN THE
UNITED STATES, 1971–72, BY AGE, RACE, AND SEX**

Race and Sex	Age 20–44	45–74
TOTAL	17.6	19.6
White Males	16.0	13.4
White Females	18.9	24.7
Black Males	10.6	7.7
Black Females	29.2	32.4

Source: 1971–72 Health and Nutrition Examination Survey, National Center for Health Statistics

who are obese is 18.9 and 24.7 for whites, while it is 29.2 and 32.4 for blacks. I feel that different eating habits account for this discrepancy and, indirectly, cause the inflated diabetes figures for nonwhites.

These unfortunate statistics are not limited to the United States. In studies investigating the number of deaths due to diabetes per 100,000 population in different countries, it was found that in no country for which there are age-adjusted statistics available do more men than women die of diabetes mellitus. As you can see from Table 3.6, quite often twice as many women die

Table 3.6

Comparison of Death Rate due to Diabetes Mellitus Age Adjusted/100,000 Population

	Year	Country	Female	Male	Ratio F/M
1.	1972	Belgium	46.8	20.3	2.31
2.	1973	Italy	30.0	16.9	1.78
3.	1974	German Dem. Rep.	25.5	11.7	2.18
4.	1970	Argentina	20.1	18.8	1.07
5.	1977	Sweden	18.8	15.4	1.22
6.	1977	Switzerland	23.2	13.9	1.67
7.	1976	U.S.A.	18.6	13.4	1.39
8.	1975	Finland	23.1	11.2	2.06
9.	1976	New Zealand	15.3	14.4	1.06
10.	1976	France	20.3	13.4	1.51
11.	1977	Australia	12.5	10.2	1.23
12.	1977	Singapore	19.9	12.9	1.54
13.	1975	Canada	15.7	12.1	1.30
14.	1977	Denmark	12.5	9.2	1.36
15.	1977	N. Ireland	4.6	3.3	1.39
16.	1974	Netherlands	13.7	7.0	1.96
17.	1977	England & Wales	11.4	8.5	1.34
18.	1976	Poland	14.3	7.5	1.91
19.	1974	Portugal	10.4	8.1	1.28
20.	1977	Japan	8.6	8.6	1.00
21.	1977	Bulgaria	11.5	9.1	1.26
22.	1977	Israel	8.1	6.9	1.17
23.	1977	Norway	9.7	7.4	1.31
24.	1977	Hungary	18.4	9.1	2.02
25.	1977	Hongkong	5.9	5.7	1.04
26.	1974	Iceland	4.7	4.6	1.02
27.	1975	Philippines	2.6	2.5	1.04
28.	1973	Trinidad	43.0	35.0	1.23
29.	1974	Luxembourg	63.0	25.0	2.52

as men. When other research related diabetic deaths to daily consumption of fat and sugar, it was hardly surprising to find that a direct correlation was found—in both post-menopausal and age-adjusted groups.

Looking at three other female groups—American, Japanese in Japan, and Japanese in Hawaii—the advantages of Westernization again come into serious question (Figure 3.1). The contrast between the native and Hawaiian Japanese destroys the "mostly heredity"

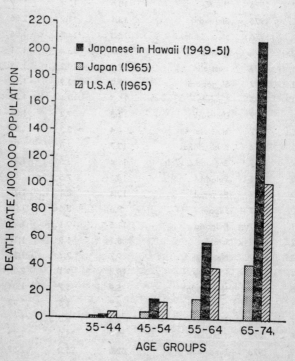

Figure 3.1

DEATH RATE IN FEMALES
DUE TO DIABETES

■ Japanese in Hawaii (1949-51)
▨ Japan (1965)
▧ U.S.A. (1965)

DEATH RATE/100,000 POPULATION

AGE GROUPS

theory of diabetes. Japanese women in Hawaii die from diabetes five times as often as Japanese women in Japan. The change to a deep-fried, high-sugar diet is the primary cause of this phenomenon.

After seeing these figures, I asked myself, very scientifically. "WHAT IN THE HELL IS GOING ON? To what crime can women attribute this punishment?" The answer *has* to be found by examining the various differences between the activities of men and women. The most obvious of these is childbearing, and so that is where I started looking.

Before the age of forty, diabetes is about as common in men as it is in women. After this age, however, as the incidence in both sexes rises, more women than men are affected. The increase in women is confined to married women; diabetes affects men and single women about equally at all ages. As the clues piled up, the finger of guilt seemed to point directly at something related to childbearing: The incidence of diabetes increases with each increase in parity (number of children).

Diabetes is twice as common in mothers of three children as in childless women, and six times as common in mothers of six or more! It seems clear that pregnancy is a potent diabetogenic stress. Some bodily changes are responsible for the greater risk of diabetes and somehow affect glucose tolerance and insulin action. Also, the increased demand on the pancreas to produce insulin during each pregnancy results in degeneration of that organ, leading to diabetes.

I believe that the change responsible for the increased risk of diabetes in women is the increase in the amount of estrogens in the body. The constant diabetogenic stress of pregnancy literally works the pancreatic islets to death. Normal women resist this stress, but women with Westernized eating habits often show an abnormal glucose tolerance test (GTT) during pregnancy. The degeneration seems to be cumulative and accounts for the progressively greater risk with each pregnancy. It is safe to say that diabetes should be taken into consideration by any woman desiring three or more children.

There are three estrogens: estrone (E1), estradiol (E2), and estriol (E3). E1 is produced primarily in obese tissues but also in the ovaries and in the adrenal glands. E2 is produced primarily in the ovaries, and some is produced in the adrenals and obese tissues. E3 is produced in the placenta during pregnancy. It is E3 in particular which contributes to enhanced insulin secretion and insulin response to glucose during pregnancy. Estriol in the blood neutralizes the effectiveness of insulin and causes the pancreas to overproduce insulin. At the same time, the blood glucose level rises, owing to the inability of the cells to use all of the sugar available. E3 increases several hundredfold during the gestation period. In pregnant diabetics, E1 and E2 are also elevated during the second half of gestation. Basically, all you need to know is that estrogens increase during pregnancy and cause cumulative diabetogenic stress.

How Estrogens Are Formed

Estrogens are formed in several ways, but in this section I will deal with the ways hormones affect women: production by the ovaries, secretion by the adrenal glands, formation by the placenta, aromatization by obese or fat tissue, and production by the intestinal bacteria. As I have said, a certain amount of estrogen in the system is normal. The estrogens produced by the ovaries, for instance, are a necessary part of the process of ovulation and reproduction. This production continues during the childbearing years and decreases after menopause. Similarly, the estrogen production by the adrenal glands and the placenta, in a healthy woman, is just part of the smooth operation of a human female body.

There are two types of estrogen production which are abnormal and under the control of the "owner" of the body—the aromatization (conversion or "making") of estrogen by adipose (fat) tissue, and the production by intestinal bacteria.

In a person of "ideal" weight, estrogens in the body taper off naturally as menopause is reached. In obese women, estrogen levels remain high and are implicated in the risk of diabetes in these women. If obese tissue is more than 50 percent of your body weight, you probably have between 2 and 5 times as much estrogen in your system as does a woman of ideal weight. For example, if your ideal weight is 100 pounds and your weight is 200, then your fat tissue is 100 pounds or 50 percent of 200. The extra estrogen in your system is what causes impaired glucose tolerance, increased insulin secretion, deterioration of pancreas function, and diabetes.

The production of estrogens by the intestinal bacteria is also under the control of the owner. When you fuel with fat, you foster the fabrication of these fecund flora. Referring to Table 3.7, we can see how in many countries (e.g., Switzerland, Sweden, the United States) the death rate from diabetes in females is related to fat and sugar intake. A diet high in fiber and complex carbohydrates speeds up your food through the intestines and prevents the overproduction of estrogens by bacteria.

Of the four ways in which estrogen is involved in women's development, I will discuss only the three in which you can exercise choice: childbearing, oral contraception, and hormone replacement therapy.

Here Lies Rabbit

It would be difficult to state a better-known fact than that there can be problems during pregnancy. The one that we are going to discuss usually does not become apparent at the time it happens, unless you are looking for it. If there is no reason to measure the expectant mother's glucose tolerance or insulin sensitivity, the problem will be missed. But it is not missed by the pancreas. When the overproduction of estrogen blocks the

31

Table 3.7

Comparison of Death Rate from Diabetes in Females with per Capita Daily Consumption of Fat and Sugar for Different Countries for 1966

	Per Capita Daily Consumption of fat & sugar gm/day	Female Death Rate/100,000 pop. (Age Adjusted)
Trinidad	159.6	23.6
German Fed. Rep.	221.2	22.6
Greece	146.0	18.6
Switzerland	259.5	23.7
Finland	226.6	18.6
France	142.6	21.2
Argentina	203.4	21.2
Sweden	248.8	20.2
U.S.A.	283.8	20.4
Hungary	187.5	13.1
Canada	281.4	14.1
New Zealand	165.0	14.5
Australia	275.3	16.9
Chile	140.2	6.1
Bulgaria	131.3	8.3
England & Wales	280.5	11.3
Portugal	126.1	9.6
Norway	251.3	7.1
Japan	92.8	6.0
Israel	204.4	4.7
Hongkong	131.8	4.0
Philippines	78.6	1.8
Taiwan	124.4	3.1

effective use of glucose in your body, and demands that the pancreas go on overtime, you will end up paying for that extra duty. With each pregnancy, the insulin "debt" increases, until the pancreas's ability to produce sufficient insulin is permanently impaired. This fact accounts for the sixfold number of deaths due to diabetes in women over forty-five who have had seven or more children. What is the message? If there is a history of diabetes in your family, and you continue to eat Westernized foods, you should seriously consider limiting your children to two.

The eating habits of the expectant mother are notorious and need reviewing. Since 90 percent of the cases of diabetes in mature women are due to diet, try not to use pregnancy as an excuse to change your eating habits—except to improve them! Your developing baby doesn't need to swim in Twinkie-fat to be healthy. On the contrary, if the baby is unusually large at birth, his/her future health is in jeopardy. Good nutrition during gestation is so important that I cannot overemphasize this point. Here is one of the few opportunities of your life in which you can actually control the future. PLEASE TAKE IT!

Did You Take Your Estrogen Today?

Do you recognize the following warnings of side effects? "You may gain or lose weight." "Your doctor may find that levels of sugar and fatty substances in your blood are elevated; the long-term effects of these changes are not known." "Other reactions . . . include . . . an increase or decrease in sex drive, appetite changes . . . If you do, you have been reading the DETAILED PATIENT LABELING in your birth-control pill package. Every warning in these inserts is there because a scientific study showed possible problems. The warnings I quoted are the ones related to diabetes and are no longer speculation.

In the years during which the pill is normally used— ages seventeen to forty-five—your body is producing estrogens in the ovaries, adrenals, placenta, intestines, and in any fat tissue you have. The last thing your body needs is an added daily "fix." True, pregnancy may also be a risk for you, but if there is a history of diabetes in your family, you should use a different method of contraception. The pill has also been connected to heart attack, destruction of vitamin B_6, depression, emotional flare-ups, irritability, fatigue, paranoia, difficulty in concentration, and sleep disturbances. Clearly your need for contraception should be balanced against the risks of these various complications in your particular case.

Birth-control pills were an overnight (literally) success when they hit the market in 1960. They became so popular so fast that their safety was tested not by laboratory animals but on the public at large (that's you!). The benefit seemed to outweigh any doubts about long-term effects. I don't have to tell the feminists that the pill was, of course, tested on women. For some reason, male "pills" need more stringent laboratory testing (?).

For every 100,000 women, between 4 and 21 die from childbirth each year, depending on age: it is not without risk. It remains more dangerous than any type of birth control until age 40, when, for smoking women on the pill, the death rate is 57 out of 100,000. The use of oral contraceptives should be considered a potent risk factor in women with metabolic disorders and avoided if possible. Traditional barrier methods backed up by abortion are from 2 to 10 times safer than any other type of contraception and from 13 to 100 times as safe as childbirth.

Bulletin: Body Facing Shutdowns in Several Areas

Suppose the kids are grown—you had only two, you are not obese, and you don't smoke. You're forty-five years old, so your body will soon be estrogen-free—right? Wrong!—if you are one of the numerous menopausal women who choose to be treated with hormone replacement therapy.

In the past, many doctors have suggested, or have been pressured into suggesting, the use of estrogen treatments for a variety of ailments, both real and imagined. Administered wisely, and in sane amounts, estrogens can be useful in the treatment of arthritis, hot flashes, sweating, bone loss, and the general softening of the figure. However, let's not forget the lessons of the previous sections in this chapter. Remember that estrogens are made in at least two other places that are still intact in your body—adipose tissue (if any) and the intestines, if your diet is high in fat and simple sugars. There is a possibility that you are still receiving a triple dose of estrogen, even though your ovaries have stopped producing it. Grodin concluded that neither adrenal nor ovarian estrogens contribute significantly to the total estrogens in the post-menopausal woman.

If you are considering estrogen therapy, please do the following: First, discuss the need and dosage with your doctor. He may not know about these new facts concerning the risk of diabetes (really!). Second, if you want the treatments, trim down your weight. There is no reason to use hormones to preserve your youth if you have already lost it to obesity. Third, during therapy restrict your intake of fat and simple sugars and increase your intake of dietary fiber. That will prevent the creation of estrogens by your intestinal bacteria.

This book and this chapter are not about dieting, but about living. Dieting, pregnancy—these are temporary conditions. Health, life—these are permanent. I am not trying to get you to go on a "two-week wonder diet," but on a lifelong health plan. First, you must determine your risk factors, such things as a family history of various diseases and your self-destructive habits. Then you must decide what you want out of life. Find out what motivates you, and use it for the will power you need to make the necessary changes. Make them gradually, or they will not be long-lasting. Eliminate one poor food and add one good one each week. Substitute skim milk for whole, margarine for butter, whole-wheat bread for white. In no time you will feel the difference—I guarantee it!

4

Modern Maturity and Diabetes

In the United States we have an abundance to eat. True, there is scattered poverty, but it only takes a trip to a really impoverished nation to realize the difference between the two levels. Americans spend well over half a trillion dollars a year in the marketplace. That market, the largest in the world, caters, of course, to consumer demand. The highest demand is for products that make life easier and reduce the effort needed to survive. The suppliers waste no time providing us with these items.

The growth of our economy depends on continuing the trend toward convenience, which in turn reduces the need for physical exertion. With countless appliances, we enjoy more leisure than any previous society. But do we spend this time on healthful activities? No. We sit mesmerized for hours by television sets that occupy 98 percent of our homes. When we do wander forth from our homes, do we walk, skate, or bicycle? Oh, sure, some do, but the majority hop into one of the several cars in the driveway. For most of us, physical effort has become a matter of choice, and it is an option we rarely take.

We are also tempted to eat more than we need. Americans spend well over $100 billion a year on food—about one-fourth of their personal income. Often rich and poor alike choose the wrong foods; the rich eat too much fat, and the poor eat too many simple carbohydrates. All of this spending attracts suppliers—close to fifty thousand today. Many of the foods that we know are unhealthy we are unable to give up because of social pressures and a tradition of their use for "hospitality." How a tradition for offering all of the worst things to our guests arose I don't know. Rather than offend them with fruit juice or carrot sticks, we tempt them with beer, potato chips, and cigarettes.

Growth in sales and income equals success in the business world. In order for the sales of food to exceed the yearly growth of the population (about 1.3 percent), the food industry realized that it needed to get us not only to eat *more* food, but also to eat *more expensive* food. The two ways to make food more expensive are to process it more and to make it more convenient to use. Sales of ready-mixed and frozen foods are growing about ten times as fast as the population. Breakfast foods, sandwich spreads, and prepared flour mixes are increasing their sales by about 8 percent a year. Virtually all of the foods experiencing such growth are either easy to prepare or edible from the package. Plain bread or coffee sales, on the other hand, increase at about the same rate as the population.

Big profits support big advertising campaigns. The food industry's $1+ billion advertising expenditure is the largest of any industry. We are assaulted by an army of "beautiful people" who swill alcohol and devour snacks, but never gain weight. We are made to feel that eating is a necessary part of all social activities and that the way to look and feel great is to "party hearty."

Low-cal and no-cal foods and beverages are sold to us at or above the price of nutritious ones. After the introduction of Diet-Rite Cola, the stock in Royal Crown Cola, the maker of Diet-Rite jumped from $7 to $43 in just a few years. It's plain to see that there is a lucrative career in appealing to the current awareness of calories and weight.

When Americans gain weight, other businesses flourish. The increasing need for oversized clothes enriches the garment and textile makers (at our expense). Every other day a new diet book (Dr. Tarnish's Silver Polish and Maraschino Cherry Miracle Two-Day Diet) is shilled. Some of these have been known to be rough on the dieter's emotional health.

Hundreds of appetite suppressants, all with the same active ingredient, are sold at outlandish prices. And the cost to the consumer for treatment of obesity and its related maladies is enormous.

The September 1980 issue of *Newsweek* reported the following figures for public spending on sickness:

1950—$12.7 billion
1980—$240 billion
1990—(projected) $758 billion

The article did not state the amount spent on prevention—virtually nothing. A drop in the ocean . . .

Reducing salons, both legitimate and bogus, attract thousands of people and their hard-earned money. Spas, gymnasiums, exercise equipment, and hot tubs are popular.

The United States is the butt of a global joke because of its citizens' growing need for enlarged seating accommodations. The Japanese invited a group of influential Americans to Tokyo to see the newly completed Olympic stadium. Unfortunately, the majority of the guests couldn't fit in the seats. When the stadium was remodeled to accommodate American posteriors, thousands of seats were lost!

Obese people wear things out faster than do trimmer folk. Shoes are squashed flat, trousers grind together between bulbous thighs, carpeting is trampled beneath nap-crushing weight, and upholstery is submitted to pressures rivaling those in a grape press. If the fat person is inactive, he or she will get caught in the vicious cycle of more weight leading to more lethargy, and so on.

The constant striving for convenience and the decreasing physical activity of Americans are two vital flaws in our way of life. These, combined with the huge financial stake business has in our gluttony, make it triply hard to follow a dietary regime. But follow we must, because of the tremendous cost of our health of doing otherwise. Americans, and members of many other cultures, eat far too much fat and sugar, and not enough fiber.

Spooning in America

When I was a kid, I naively believed my friends when they told me that I would get "sugar diabetes" if I ate too much sugar. Ha! Later I heard that it was hereditary and was *so* relieved. Unfortunately, it can now be shown that sugar abuse and its result, obesity, definitely lead to diabetes.

Every morning each person gets 100 "percents" to spend on calories. Whether you end up eating 5,000 calories or 1,200, they still are 100 percent of your calories for that day. In the United States, each person spends 15 to 25 "percents" on sugar; 32 teaspoons a day—125 pounds a year. Since your mental calculator is now whirring, trying somehow to prove me wrong, let's look at the sugar content of some of our favorite foods. There are 7 teaspoons of sugar in 12 ounces of cola or other soft drinks. That's almost one-fourth of the daily amount right there. A slice of chocolate cake has 10 teaspoons, 4 ounces of hard candy has 20, a tablespoon of jelly has 4.6, and a slice of berry pie has 10. If you have the nerve to read the labels on the packaged foods you eat, you'll find much more.

Sugar, since it has no nutrients of its own, robs your system of the ones it needs to be digested. What alternatives are there to sugar? Some health food stores will try to tell you that brown sugar is superior to the white, refined kind, but the truth of the matter is that brown sugar, despite its traces of nutrients, is little better than white. Honey, while still not very nutritious, is fructose and must be processed by the liver before it gets into the bloodstream. Therefore it doesn't cause the tremendous jump in blood sugar level that sucrose causes. Maple syrup and molasses are even slightly better than honey. They have more of the nutrients that are needed for their own digestion. All of these substitutes are still sugar and must be counted as such when you are figuring out your intake of sugar.

Many people, even some athletic coaches, mistakenly believe that your blood must have the sugar content of blackstrap or you won't have energy. On the contrary, you need only two teaspoons of glucose in your bloodstream at any given time. While it's true that simple sugars, being easy to digest, get into the blood sooner than protein, their effect is short-lived. All foods get changed to glucose in the body and therefore can be used to provide energy. If for some reason an athlete has depleted his energy, a bit of honey or fruit is fine to use for a pick-me-up, but it is not meant to replace solid nutrition.

It is true that our bodies burn food, because the glucose circulating through our system is oxidized—a type of burning. The process of oxidation takes certain nutrients. Some food companies seem to think that nature made mistakes on many of its products, and have set about improving them. What usually happens is that a perfect food is ruined by man's meddling. For instance, oranges contain all the nutrients needed for their own digestion; none need to be stolen from the body. Table sugar, on the other hand, increases your need for vitamins by using more than its share.

Fat's on!

Let's say that you've spent 20 "percents" of your 100 on sugar. Of the remaining 80, the average American will spend about 40 more on fat. Suppose the boss is coming over and you want to serve him a typical "com-

41

pany meal." The menu usually looks something like this:

Cocktails with cheese dip	91% fat
Potato chips	63% fat
Avocado with mayonnaise	90% + 100% fat
Porterhouse steak	82% fat
with butter	100% fat
French fries	44% fat
Salad—lettuce	0%
with Italian dressing	97% fat
Old-fashioned pound cake	56% fat
with ice cream	65% fat

Total—79% fat, 5,000 calories. Twice as many as you need for a whole day!

Where is fat hidden? Basically, fat comes from animal and vegetable sources. We get animal fat from beef, pork, other meats, milk (cream, cheese, butter), and poultry. Vegetable fats are found in the various oils made from nuts, seeds, and grains. Fats can be either saturated or unsaturated. Saturated fats, the ones to restrict, are usually solid at room temperature, while unsaturated ones are usually liquid. Hydrogenated is another word for saturated. You need only about 20 to 25 percent of your calories from fat. A healthy balance of calories would be: carbohydrates—60 percent; protein—15 percent; and fat—25 percent. Carbohydrate consumption should be divided into complex carbohydrate—45 percent—and simple—15 percent.

So Refined

The word "refined" may have a very good connotation when used to describe a person's character or personality, but its virtuous reputation should not cloud its sinister relationship to food and nutrition. Before much was known about health, the process of refining various products was discovered and used to solve some of the numerous problems of nineteenth-century food distribution and use. In the days before refrigeration and mechanical transportation, the time from the harvesting of food to its consumption was quite long. Whole wheat, among other things, would not store for long at room temperatures. Someone discovered that if the germ and bran were removed from the freshly harvested wheat, it would neither spoil nor attract insects. (That makes sense—refined flour will not sustain insect, animal, *or* human life.) Twenty-two (!) nutrients were, for forty or more years, stripped from the wheat. In 1930, the government decided that refined flour should contain something, so it required the mills to replace *four* of the missing twenty-two. The refiners, of course, picked the four cheapest ones and locked them into chemical compounds which the body's digestive systems cannot break down. The only real bread we have enjoyed since 1900 was during the two wars, when the milling ratio was changed to accommodate the war effort. Both times the diabetes rate decreased markedly in all countries where wheat germ and bran were left in the bread for military reasons! (See Figure 2.3.)

When there is little or no fiber in your diet, your digestion suffers. Your intestines need something to stimulate peristalsis (the squeezing action of the intestine). Fiber provides this bulk. Eating fiber can help cut down on calories, for it gives a full feeling without adding more calories to the diet. With fiber in the diet you can avoid constipation, speed up digestion, inhibit harmful intestinal bacteria, and lower the risk of cancer of the colon, diverticulosis, varicose veins, and heart disease.

The Funafuti Study

Funafuti is the main island of Tuvalu, a group of Polynesian islands in the Central Pacific. Until about thirty years ago, the inhabitants of these islands enjoyed

43

a communal lifestyle and lived on a diet consisting almost exclusively of products found on the island: fish, coconut, breadfruit, plantains (bananas), and taro (roots).

In 1942, the U.S. Navy established an air base there and relocated some of the natives. To repay them for this inconvenience, packaged flour, rice, sugar, and other foodstuffs were brought in, and the Funafutians began to depend on these sources of "nourishment." The practice continued after the war, and now 80 percent of the food used on the island is provided by a food cooperative set up in 1948.

In a study conducted by Wicking et al., 110 adult Funafutians were given a blood glucose test and a dietary survey. It was found that they eat 33 percent of their calories in fat; women have twice the diabetes prevalence of men; diabetes, previously rare, is now 11 percent, and hypertension is 11 percent. What happened here is a classic instance of dietary Westernization. Polynesians have a strong predisposition for diabetes, but don't normally get the disease. Hypertension is unknown in the outer islands, where the diet has not changed. The researchers conclude: "From these studies there is evidence to implicate the change from traditional to Western lifestyle as a major factor in the increase in diabetes prevalence. Obesity, decreased physical activity, and a high-calorie, refined carbohydrate diet are possible major culprits in this change."

It is still possible to live off local foods in Funafuti and other Polynesian islands, but the convenience of the packaged flour, sugar, rice, canned fish, meat, fruits and vegetables, soft drinks, and beer has caused the natives to switch to these. The imported diet is particularly low in protein, vitamins, minerals, and fiber. The authors of the study state: "Marked obesity is now a characteristic of many Micronesian and Polynesian populations, and must rank as a major causative factor for the diabetes and hypertension explosion."

The kind of diet most Americans (and many other folks, including Funafutians) eat is incompatible with the biochemical makeup of a human being. Whether or not you are getting the right nutrients can be determined by a blood or hair analysis. Our bodies, while they do not always show the effects of abuse immediately, are delicate and can be seriously disrupted by even the slightest imbalance in chemistry. One cola beverage, for instance, upsets the calcium and phosporous levels in your system for twelve to twenty-four hours and can inhibit the action of the white blood cells for the same period. When you load your system with simple sugars, your liver and pancreas get confused by the abnormal amount of demand placed on them. They can degenerate over time.

When you eat complex carbohydrates, insulin requirements are more even, and the liver has a much easier time maintaining the proper blood-sugar level. You are less likely to experience behavior problems, allergies, emotional difficulties, and impaired defenses to disease. But if you start your day with sweet rolls and coffee, by midmorning your quick energy burst has been drowned in insulin. When the snack wagon comes around, you'll be tempted to eat the fast digesting treats it offers—usually the same thing you had for breakfast. The cycle continues all day as you and your pancreas get the workout of your lives. The result is that you are hungry and irritable all day. The sad part is that you start accepting the way you feel as normal or inevitable, when it could easily be reversed.

You may have seen something similar to what I saw while on a flight to Arizona. Two friends of mine, both physicians, and I were enjoying the precocious and clever antics of a young black boy about ten years old. He was talkative, without being bothersome, and had a good sense of humor. About a half an hour before landing, his mother reached into her purse and gave junior a candy bar she had been saving for the end of the journey. Within minutes, what had been a very entertaining young gentleman became a disagreeable, squalling brat, who proceeded to squirm, kick, and fidget his way out of our hearts as quickly and easily as he had charmed his way into them in the first place. I urge you, if you have children who are sometimes hyperactive, keep a chart of their food intake and any behavior problems for one month. In this way, correlations will show up and can be corrected.

There are other more serious consequences of improper diet than hyperactivity. Heart attack, hypertension, diabetes, and cancer have all been connected to bad eating habits.

The dangers of poor diet are not all physical. By not watching your eating habits, you can become susceptible to numerous mental disorders as well. You age sooner and are hospitalized with no "organic" cause; you may look O.K., but inside you are not. Dr. E. Cheraskin, and Dr. W. M. Ringsdorf, Jr., in their fine book *Psychodietetics* describe in detail the relationship between food and mood. They say that since the brain is an organ, it needs constant and balanced nutrition, just like any other organ. Poor diet leads to metabolic distortion and therefore can cause tension, nervousness, anxiety, the jitters, overweight, or fatigue. Metabolic imbalance has even been implicated in schizophrenia, alcoholism, drug dependency, psychosis, and depression.

There are twenty million Americans headed for a breakdown. Quite often, persons who are unhappily married are really suffering from dietary deficiencies, not social incompatibilities. Dr. Cecelia Rosenfeld has found that "in a surprising number of broken marriages, spouses suffered from a blood-sugar imbalance." Dr. Donald Eccleston found that biochemical lesions can cause moods. Other studies have linked diet to crime, car accidents, sex problems, learning disability, juvenile delinquency, behavior problems, and senility.

It is amazing to remember that we didn't know what

caused *any* disease until the discovery, in 1865, of germs. Now that we have conquered most of the contagious diseases, it is high time we paid some attention to our new problem—the degenerative diseases. Just as it is true that three people, all exposed to a common cold, will not always get the same severity of symptoms, people react to deficient diets in different ways. These "psychic germs," as Cheraskin and Ringsdorf call nutrient deficiencies, will break down your body's defenses and cause different symptoms in each individual.

Fifty years ago the Germans discovered psychosomatics and established that emotions can alter endocrine balance and impede digestion. Is it any wonder, then, that the reverse is true? When your diet is lacking in important nutrients, your resistance to disease—mental as well as physical—is lowered.

The Diet Doldrums

One of the main reasons people go off their diets is that they don't seem to feel as good on the diet as they did before. The reason is not that being thin is painful, but that most diets are too drastic and deficient in nutrients. Don't *ever* eat fewer than 600 calories a day unless you are under 24-hour supervision by a physician. Your brain alone needs this amount just to regulate your bodily functions properly. A much better daily minimum would be about 1,200 calories, because only a trained dietitian can squeeze all of your needs into fewer. If you try to lose too fast and don't get a balanced diet, it can actually affect your sanity!

If you're still wondering whether to diet, let me point out some of the problems of the obese.

> 96% have digestive problems.
> 37% have an abnormal glucose tolerance.
> 28% have poor protein metabolism.
> 73% have poor fat metabolism.
> 18% have abnormal basal metabolism.

Abnormal basal metabolism is the *result*, not the cause of obesity.

47

If you have any kind of problem that is not responding to ordinary curative measures, find a responsible doctor to help you investigate the trouble from a nutritional point of view. It does not matter whether the problem is physical or mental. Even if it seems entirely unrelated to food, do not make a hasty judgment. If the symptoms are sexual in nature, there is a very good possibility that nutrition would help. While there is no magical aphrodisiac, many foods contain elements crucial to proper functioning of the sex organs.

Senility is not an inevitability of old age. It is the slowing down of brain functions because of decreased circulation and lack of certain vital chemicals. It does not have to happen! It has been successfully treated with vitamins.

Food allergies, of course, respond to regulating the intake of the offending substance. Often, though, the victim will crave the very thing that irritates him or her. You can use a simple pulse test to determine if a food bothers you. Compare your normal pulse with your pulse after eating a suspected food. If it is high, try eliminating the food for a week to see if the condition goes away.

The modern world is full of wonderful opportunities and carefully concealed deathtraps. We cannot go wandering through the supermarket nibbling indiscriminately like two-legged goats, hoping that what we eat will be what we need. The right of choice demands the use of carefully collected facts to arrive at an intelligent decision. I know that some readers will claim that the body "tells" them what to eat, and thereby justify everything they eat as beneficial. That might have been true when the selection only included those foods provided by nature. But man has befuddled that old system beyond fixing. There are too many poor choices available. Every person whose daily routine requires him to select food, for himself or others, *must* learn nutrition to survive.

5

Obesity, Diabetes, and Altered Sexual Awareness

Theodore B. Van Itallie, in his excellent article "Dietary Fiber and Obesity," published in the *American Journal of Clinical Nutrition,* 1978, states that obesity is "the most common form of malnutrition in the United States and in many other foreign countries." He feels that the two main reasons for this surprising fact are diet and level of physical activity. As we saw in the previous chapter, modern machines have reduced effort for many Americans, both at home and on the job. Supermarkets make shopping easier, and high-powered promotions force our hand at the store.

Reducing effort reduces the number of calories necessary in our diet. Unfortunately, folks, all that mental stress you put up with at work doesn't burn one single calorie. It does do other things, which we'll discuss later. The sedentary lifestyle we now "enjoy" demands lighter eating.

We have behaved as if the opposite were true. Since 1889 we have increased our consumption of fats and simple sugars and decreased our intake of complex carbohydrates, which provide beneficial dietary fiber. The process of refining has stolen all the benefits from the food and made it more calorie-concentrated. Fiber in food is beneficial for several reasons: it promotes chewing and increases the effort needed to eat; it reduces the rate of eating; it decreases the absorption of food in the intestines; it adds heartiness to food, making it more filling; and it seems to prevent obesity in populations

49

eating a high-fiber diet. Animals that normally eat a high-fiber diet become obese when put on a diet of refined food. Fiber also stimulates the secretion of saliva and gastric juices, which help fill the stomach. A diet high in fiber can truly lead to weight loss.

Obese people will eat less if forced to work to obtain food. In one study, subjects were divided into obese and lean subgroups. As both groups' attention was focused elsewhere, nuts were provided as a snack. Sometimes the nuts were in the shells, and at other times the nuts were without shells. About half of the lean subjects ate nuts, and it did not matter whether the nuts were in the shells or not. Obese subjects always ate the nuts without the shells, but only one in twenty ate nuts when they had to shell them. In another study, milkshakes were offered with either a big-bore or a small-bore straw. Lean subjects drank about the same amount of milkshake through each straw, but obese subjects drank much more through the "easy" straw than through the "difficult" straw. In the same way, by processing the fiber out of food, we make it easy for people to overeat, and difficult for them to reduce.

I know that you are tired of hearing about laboratory rats, but I cannot resist the temptation to tell you about two types used in experiments concerning obesity: the Zucker "fat rat" and the Sclafani and Springer "dietary-obese rat." The Zucker rat becomes obese when given unlimited access to standard rat pellets. These pellets are nutritious but ordinary. When examined, Zucker rats show not only bigger fat cells, but *more* fat cells than other rats. These rats are genetically obese.

The Sclafani rat is a dietary-obese rat. It too gains weight, but only if offered snack foods along with the rat pellets. Such things as chocolate, candy bars, marshmallows, cookies, bananas, salami, cheese, and sugared breakfast food, when added to the diet, produced obesity. When these things were withdrawn, the rats reduced their eating until their weight was normal. While not all rats gained equally, most became obese on the junk-food diet.

Two types of obesity, similar to the types found in the rat models, have been distinguished in humans. In one type the fat cells are bigger and more numerous than in lean subjects, and in the other they are just bigger. I feel that genetic obesity in humans is caused by overnutrition during gestation and infant years, while the dietary type is caused by a Westernized high-fat, high-sugar, low-fiber diet. Both can lead to diabetes, and both can be reversed, but the person with genetic obesity will need to follow a more stringent diet than his dietary-obese neighbor.

The curious reader may at this point wonder why, if to gain weight is unhealthy, the body has the ability to do so. Good question. Margaret J. Albrink, in her paper "Cultural and Endocrine Origins of Obesity," says, "A genetic tendency to conserve calories as fat might have been . . . useful when calories were scarce, but would lead to obesity in a society where food is plentiful." She also blames massive advertising for our "desire for . . . sedentary, effortless, overfed existance."

I think it's clear that the United States and certain other Westernized countries are dangerous places to live from a dietary point of view. Obesity is hard to avoid here, and so the consequences of obesity need to be made known.

Fat and Insulin

The evidence for a connection between obesity and diabetes, atherosclerosis, and hypertension is too conclusive to ignore. Obesity and atherosclerosis, for example, are so common among middle-aged persons that it is difficult to find subjects without either ailment to use in a study of the relationship. But in the studies that have been done, a single fact was of central importance— obesity increases the blood concentration of insulin.

Insulin is produced in the pancreas. Any increase in insulin production means that the pancreas is working harder than usual to make it. As with the heart, any time a body organ is chronically forced to increase its workload, certain changes take place in that organ. In the case of the pancreas, the beta cells, which produce the insulin, increase in number and output. This strain is a potent diabetogenic stress and leads to diabetes.

Excess insulin is the *result,* not the cause of obesity. Not only does overeating stimulate insulin production, but weight gain causes your system to become resistant to insulin—more and more is required. Eventually your pancreas gets confused and worn out, and diabetes results.

Abnormalities of insulin production and glucose tolerance are measured in several ways. The oral glucose tolerance test (OGTT) measures how your body reacts to the eating of a specific amount of sugar. Fat people usually cannot use blood sugar as quickly and easily as leaner ones. Their blood-sugar level stays higher for a longer time than normal.

The level of insulin in the blood is another way of testing for an abnormal metabolism. Obese persons show an increased amount of insulin circulating in the bloodstream. When both glucose intolerance and hyperinsulinism are found together, that is evidence of insulin resistance in the tissues, because in a normal person the presence of glucose and insulin in the blood would lead to glucose use by the tissues.

When the pancreas is in a constant state of overuse, it is also much more influenced by stress. The secretion of insulin is under three types of control: blood contents, hormones, and brain signals. It is the connection with the brain and hormones that makes the pancreas susceptible to stress and which, in turn, makes stress a factor in diabetes.

I should mention here that chronic use of alcohol is dangerous in conjunction with obesity. Alcohol is very similar to sugar from a chemical standpoint. This means that it is very easy to digest and is a potent stimulator of the pancreas. Also, it overworks the liver and can lead to various liver ailments. Since the liver is responsible for processing unwanted products in the body, its ability to rid the body of estrogens is impaired. We'll see why that is important later.

Proof of the fact that obesity *causes* increased insulin production, and not the other way around, is good news because that means when obese persons with hyperinsulinemia reduce their weight, the symptoms go away. Another important clue is that a diet high in complex carbohydrates helps correct the problem. Of course, increased weight gain and high fat-sugar diet make the condition worse.

Insulin Resistance

To quote again from Dr. Albrink: "Hyperinsulinism reflects a compensatory adaptation to some insulin-antagonizing force. . . . Agents that impair glucose metabolism and cause a compensatory increase in insulin may cause obesity." In other words the body adapts to an inability to use insulin by making more of it; this makes you fat. This resistance showed up in study subjects who volunteered to overeat and become fat. Again, when they reduced, the condition went away. Another researcher found that the amount of insulin resistance was in proportion to the amount of fat tissue.

What is the implication of all this? We are going to show that the cause of insulin resistance is the sex hormone estrogen. We will show that estrogen affects the pancreas, the liver, the kidneys, the fat and muscle tissue, the sex organs, and two important parts of the central nervous system.

I would like to make an analogy between the estrogen in your system and a lost flock of proliferous pigeons.

Figure 5.1

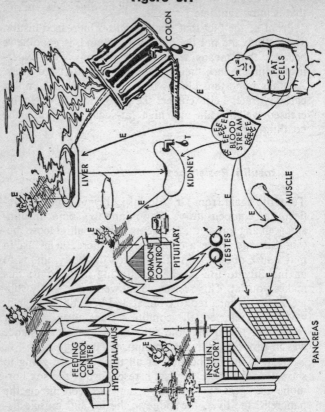

Making use of the diagram (Figure 5.1), picture your internal organs as a network of interrelated buildings and machines, much as in a small town. Various products circulate in the economy, as do television signals, which instruct the workers in each building about the day's work. When these signals arrive clearly and on time, the work is accomplished with ease and efficiency. But when estrogens circulate through your system, it is as if a flock of birds is perched on the antennae of your telecommunication set. Signals either can't get through at all or are hopelessly botched by the time they arrive. These signals affect your digestive, endocrine, nervous, and reproductive systems.

Estrogens produced in the intestines by bacteria travel to the liver by way of the circulation between the two. The liver tries to deactivate (conjugate) these and send them back for further digestion, but the bacteria merely reactivate them. This starts one flock of "birds" through your system. Fat tissue, also a source of birds, dumps estrogen into the bloodstream, and this flock nests anywhere blood goes: the liver, kidney, muscles, pancreas, and brain. Special antennae in the hypothalamus, pituitary, and liver are favorite perches. Estrogen in these areas blocks the reception of important instructions in various organs. The kidneys start clearing the body of male hormones. The eating center (hypothalamus) thinks the body is too thin and signals for overeating behavior. The pituitary, which controls the sex glands, is not alerted to the drastically low levels of male hormone in men and therefore does not order more to be made. Even the brain's stress center is constantly stimulated, and eating seems to ease the uncomfortable feeling temporarily. The effects of estrogen excess are different in men and women, so I will discuss each one separately.

Guys

Impotence is a rather frequent symptom in obese or diabetic patients. This phenomenon has been traced to the low levels of unbound testosterone in their blood. When estrogens are made in the intestine and in fat tissue, they circulate through the system and confuse other organs. The liver, for instance, is supposed to create sex-hormone-binding-globulin (SHBG). Estrogens prevent the formation of SHBG and cause male hormones to be excreted instead of retained in the body. This lowers the concentration of testosterone in the blood. When a man has less testosterone, his sex drive is lowered. Also, normally the pituitary, sensing the need for testosterone, would signal the testes to make more. "Birds" ruin this line of communication, and the testes never get the message. (You get it, though, because you wonder why the honeymoon has ended—never realizing it's your added weight or faulty diet that is the problem.)

You have already read how obesity causes increased insulin production. Studies have shown that as the amount of insulin in the blood is increased, the urinary production rate of estrogens is also increased, proving a relationship between the two. Oddly, there are no exterior sex signs of feminization which accompany this type of hormonal imbalance, which is the reason why researchers missed this important discovery for so long.

At virtually every seminar I give, nationwide, several men linger after the end of the session. If given the chance to talk to me alone, they tell me the sad tale of a marriage on the rocks. They are baffled. They have sought all kinds of professional help. They have been told that their condition is "normal." They have been told that it is "all in their heads." Some have even been to astrologers and fortune tellers, but the answer will not be found in the occult.

I ask them about their youth. How much did they weigh when they were nineteen? What were their eating habits? They shake their heads. They start to understand that a human body performs according to how it's treated. It is a scientific fact that your sex life needn't be all downhill after age forty. It is dragged down by the general state of your health. Dr. Paul Carpenter, a Mayo Clinic specialist in endocrinology, in an Associated Press story, "Man's sex drive 'not all downhill' after 40" (Columbus *Dispatch*, March 22, 1981), says that while "studies done 30 years ago indicated the male sex drive, libido and potency, decline as levels of the testosterone hormone diminish with advancing age, more recent studies say this may not be the case."

It seems that the earlier studies were done at hospitals, and the health of the subjects is now in question. Carpenter states that men who are otherwise healthy maintain their sex drive into advanced years, based on the amount of testosterone still in their system.

I totally agree. There is absolutely no inevitability to the loss of sex drive in the human male. By eating poorly and getting fat, we are drowning our testosterone in a sea of female hormones. If you want to do something about it, you can. Chapter 8 will deal with the treatment and reversal of these problems.

Gals

All the nasty things that estrogens do to men are a problem with women too, except that in one area the effect is the opposite. Since you are female, estrogen is "your hormone." What is causing hubby's lack of interest is causing an increased need for love and affection in you. Since a couple normally eat the same foods, they often get obese together. But that is where "together" ends, because her increased urge is met with his increased indifference. I'm so absolutely convinced that this problem is very widespread in our society that I consider this chapter to be one of the most important.

When your fat tissue and intestinal bacteria produce estrogens, the same things happen to your metabolic system that happen to a man's. "Birds" confuse the instructions to and from the eating center and the pancreas. Too much insulin is produced, an insulin resistance occurs in the cells, and blood sugar cannot be effectively used. The increased stress put on the pancreas leads to diabetes.

As I said in Chapter 3, women have several extra sources of estrogens that men don't have. Every time a female is pregnant, the excess estrogen in her system insults an already busy pancreas. After three children, a woman's chances of getting diabetes are increased by the birth of each successive child. Women who have had six or more children are high diabetes risks.

The extra estrogens produced by fat tissue and in the intestines are sometimes added to by the use of birth-control pills and post-menopausal estrogen treatments.

Any extra estrogen in your system increases the insulin resistance of your tissues and raises the risk of diabetes. Again, please weigh the benefits of these treatments against the dangers before deciding to use them.

The Hypothalamus

The hypothalamus is part of the central nervous system (brain). We need to discuss it briefly because it has been proved to have three functions related to diabetes. The hypothalamus, or eating center, emits signals that control insulin level and eating. Also found there is a stress center. Two parts of this organ have opposite functions.

Figure 5.2

		insulin	you feel	stress
ventral medial hypothalamus	if stimulated	decreases	full	is lowered
	if impaired	increases	hungry	is raised
ventral lateral hypothalamus	if stimulated	increases	hungry	is raised
	if impaired	decreases	full	is lowered

If all these things are controlled by the feeding center, then it follows that information necessary for making these decisions must be received by it. Also, if insulin is controlled by the hypothalamus, there must be a line of communication between it and the pancreas. Both of these deductions are true. But, as you have already seen, estrogens block the receiving mechanisms of the hypothalamus. Thus, the signals it sends to other organs are scrambled. From Figure 5.2 you can see that when insulin is high, you feel hungry. When there are estrogens in your system and a resistance to insulin in the tissues, you tend to eat more than you need, because the food can't be used by the body. The estrogens block the feeding center's "full" signals.

Studies have shown that insulin causes animals to eat. Other studies showed that increasing doses of insulin caused overweight. The cutting of the nerve from the hypothalamus to the pancreas reversed the weight gain caused by the destruction of hypothalamus receptors, unless the animal was on a high-fat diet.

These facts prove a strong connection between the hypothalamus and obesity and diabetes. The more estrogen in your system, the more receptive the feeding center is to it, and the more insulin will be produced—causing degeneration of the pancreas.

There is also a connection between the hypothalamus and production of male hormone in men. In a normal subject, the hypothalamus tests the blood and signals the pituitary concerning the amounts of testosterone. When the hypothalamus's estrogen receptors are blocked, a false signal tells the pituitary that testosterone levels are fine, when in reality they are low compared to estrogen. This is what causes the lowered sexual interest in males eating a high fat diet and carrying excess weight.

Finally, the hypothalamus controls the "sex" of the liver. Yes, you read correctly. You see, the liver is a sort of filter. Among its functions, it tries to rid the body of "opposite sex" hormones. In men, the liver filters out estrogen, and in women, testosterone. The pituitary actually controls the "sex" of the liver in women by emitting a "feminizing factor." In men, the hypothalamus prevents this by releasing a "feminizing-factor-release-inhibiting-factor." Thoroughly confused? When the man's hypothalamus is blocked by estrogen, it allows the pituitary to feminize the liver. The liver then starts to clear out *male* hormone from the man! Now do you see that a feminized liver is undesirable? This is precisely why a man can have lots of estrogen in his system without the body trying to get rid of it. This allows diabetes to develop over time, because of high insulin levels, glucose *in*tolerance, insulin resistance in the tissues, and resultant wearing out of the pancreas.

In this chapter I have shown you how obesity leads

to insulin production, diabetes, and altered sexual awareness. When men have too much estrogen, their urge is lowered; when women have too much estrogen, their urge is higher. In Chapter 8 I will tell how these conditions can be *totally reversed*!

Human Stories: Kathryn

This is the story of Kathryn. The medical and psychological facts are precisely preserved and concern an actual person. The names, family constellations, and all other details are completely fabricated to protect the confidentiality in which the information was given.

Kathryn

I was raised in a very strict religious environment. My father believed that if you had sinful thoughts, it was the same as sinning. Sex was never mentioned.

I met my husband during my senior year in college, and we were married. He was good-looking, not obese, but never thin. I desired sex much more than he did, and became the assertive one.

I had my first child by Caesarian section, then four years later a second, and a third in rapid succession. I was very oversexed during this period.

We decided to have my tubes tied, but this destroyed my motivation to be the assertive one in sex. I waited for my husband to take over this role, but he never did.

I was gaining more weight and went to a doctor for diet pills. These, along with family pressures, nearly put me over the edge. Since our sex life hadn't improved, I decided to have a "heart-to-heart" with my husband. This resulted in making an appointment with a sex therapist.

We attended sessions for some time, but there was no improvement. We saw the therapist separately for a while, but when I asked him why there was no change in my husband, he pleaded patient confidentiality! Dead end. I told my husband he could quit therapy, but that I would no longer be the aggressor in sex. I felt that because I was heavy, I was no longer desirable.

Soon my husband had a massive coronary, brought on by the flu. He tried to satisfy me with a vibrator for a while, but I didn't enjoy this type of lovemaking, preferring masturbation.

After my husband's coronary he was diagnosed diabetic and was quite overweight. I would prepare his special diet, but he would sabotage the regimen by sneaking sweets at other times of the day. He was forced to retire at age 46. Even though I weighed 255, I entered the job market.

I was also taking classes in psychology, where the instructor suggested that I lose weight to improve my self-esteem. This advice from a stranger motivated me to do just that, and the pounds melted away.

I met an interesting man during the course of some assigned research projects in psychology and felt that I was becoming attracted to him.

My conscience bothered me, but soon the friendship developed into a full-blown affair, my need for sex winning out over my religious upbringing. My husband was completely impotent during the early months of my affair and died after one year.

I can't express the anguish that my sexual incompatibility with my husband caused me. I had to change my whole value system—at no small cost. But I know that there are many women like me out there. I advise them to get either a divorce or a lover. Having an affair saved my sanity and changed my life.

Comment

Kathryn's story has three important parts: the upbringing of the characters, the effects of obesity and health on their marriage, and the painful changes in this woman's value system brought on by the conflict between the first two factors.

My research has shown a definite relationship between obesity and sexual drive. Sadly, this effect is not the same in men as it is in women. Sex urge is regulated by the levels of hormones in the body—testosterone for men, estrogen for women. We have discovered that estrogens are produced in two previously misunderstood ways. They are produced in the intestines by the microflora or bacteria which flourish there because of improper diet, and they are actually produced by adipose or fat tissue itself. This double-whammy of estrogen production is characterized in females by exaggerated sex urge and in men by lowered sex drive. Both conditions reinforce themselves in a vicious circle. As her urge grows and isn't fulfilled, she may eat more to comfort herself or to protect herself from extramarital temptation. He may also eat because food is the only source of pleasure that remains. What results is a couple that started out with minor differences and ends up totally incompatible, and unhealthy to boot!

The conflict, as in Kathryn's case, arises when the female's physical needs overwhelm her religious upbringing and she strays from the marital bed. This type of pressure is very powerful and can be destructive to all concerned. My mission is to spread the knowledge of how diet affects sexual drive so that you, the reader, can better understand what is going on in our food-oriented society and possibly in your family.

6

Sexuality in Obesity and Diabetes: Case Histories

Maria Simonson, Sc.D., Ph.D.,
Johns Hopkins Hospital, Baltimore, Md.

What makes us want to eat? We eat because we see food. We smell it cooking and hear it cooking. We remember the taste of food and recall the texture. Also, food is simply available. But food can often be a tranquilizer—a substitute for love and affection. A patient of mine once said, "My stomach doesn't know the difference between love and food."

Marital problems often cause this non-nutritional need for food. More women than men have this need. Many things could contribute to the use of food as a substitute for love—loneliness, rejection, a mundane job, pressures, sexual dissatisfaction, delayed maturation. A regression to infantile gratifications can result in an attempt to alleviate anxieties, tensions, anger, and frustrations by overeating. Food is one form of attention you can give yourself, so overeating should be recognized as a symbol of unfulfilled needs in other areas of life: intellectual, sexual, social, and financial. If you add to overeating the additional problem of daydreaming and its low energy expenditure, you get a resultant weight gain.

Another cause of obesity is what we call "diet anger"—the desire to punish oneself for one's feelings or actions. Eating can also be a barrier against undesired contact or activity. A person can use obesity as an excuse not to participate in some aspects of marriage, such as sex and parenthood, or aspects of society—work, community affairs, or social activities.

Often, when people are using their weight as a barrier, forced reducing can produce psychosis; the weight was a necessary adaptation. So we find that, for some, obesity is actually attractive. Using fatness as a weapon of offense, as well as defense, is sometimes the only form of adaption these people are able to make to certain lifestyles and situations. Some people actually perform better with a little weight on them, because their body image is threatened by weight loss. A person who "throws his weight around" or makes "weighty decisions" or whose arguments "carry a lot of weight" may feel that physical size is a symbol of power. Unfortunately, fat is neither powerful nor healthy, and certainly not sexy!

Being overweight can affect your sex life. The danger with pseudopsychologists and weight-loss quacks is that they do not know or treat the true reasons for this serious side effect of obesity. To treat the obese person who has libido problems one must, after evaluation and consultation, get his weight down. In the majority of cases, the added weight causes endocrine and hormonal problems which negatively affect the sex drive. A lack of sex can destroy any relationship.

Several other related problems are worth mentioning. Obesity can cause irregular menstrual periods. During the later childbearing years, the fear of pregnancy is a big enough problem, but if it is further complicated month-to-month, it is much worse. Another problem for the obese person can be the slim friend or sister, whose company always ends up a bad influence and source of stress.

Lack of sex hormones is related to many cases of obesity. We had a young obese boy in our clinic whose problem seemed to be hormonal, and after a change in eating regimen and reexamination, the tests showed a very different hormonal pattern and metabolic rate.

Less than 6 percent of obesity, however, is *caused* by glandular problems.

Another type we often see is the obese body-builder type who has very accentuated muscle development, hypervirilism, and boundless energy. People of this type have a tremendous appetite, and their obesity, usually in the trunk, neck, and face, is of great proportions. Others with Cushing's disease, Frohlich's disease, or gonadal obesity show a decreased libido—some without external changes.

Let's look at the case of Dorothy, an overweight twenty-nine-year-old housewife. She had started to feel that, because of her weight gain, her husband didn't love or understand her. There was a lack of communication. He would nag her about her weight, and she would eat more to pacify her hurt feelings. She had high blood sugar and insulin insensitivity. She was uncooperative at our diabetic clinic because she felt she deserved the punishment of rejection for her crime of fatness. Before we could reduce her, we had to treat her psychologically. After counseling, she was put on a diet and lost 112 pounds. Her blood sugar and glucose tolerance returned to normal. Her husband is still a problem, but, as is often the case, he will not agree to counseling or accept any blame.

Ruth was quite obese, and her relationship with a married man was unsatisfactory sexually and psychologically. She perceived the death of her father as a punishment for her immoral relationship. Guilt caused her to pressure her lover to get a divorce and marry her, and it also caused her to eat. He found these new behaviors unattractive and broke up with her. As she ate more and became depressed, she entered into a series of promiscuous relationships in which she was used as a sex object by uncaring men. In therapy she learned that she was punishing herself. Now, with slow progress, she has changed her behavior and lost weight, but her guilt remains.

Michael was thirty-six years old when he came to see

us, and was sixty-three pounds overweight. He had been gaining more and more weight and had experienced a diminishing sex drive. His marriage had been normal, but after his divorce he had experienced more than the normal decrease in sexual interest. His heterosexual activities were so infrequent that he was approached by a homosexual acquaintance. Afraid that he harbored dormant homosexual tendencies, he came to us to see if the weight gain was a manifestation of this. He was counseled, tested, and put on a diet. In seven and a half months he lost weight, and his sex drive returned to normal.

Kathy was twenty-four years old and overweight. She was overly demonstrative and affectionate, so much so that she drove men away with her sexual overtures. She resented her thin friends at work, and became promiscuous in an attempt to prove herself more attractive than they. She ate to compensate for her anger toward her colleagues. She went to a weight-loss franchise and lost a considerable amount of weight, despite the high cost and unprofessional treatment. As she became obsessed with dieting, her sexual urges decreased and were replaced by anorexic desires. Sex became unimportant, where once it had been all-consuming. She is now under psychiatric care.

Marjorie was a passive type who never expressed her normal anger and resentments. Her husband was a disagreeable, criticizing man. His constant nagging caused her overeating. A vicious circle of ridicule and weight gain ensued. She was aware that her overeating was psychological in origin, and she punished her husband by denying him sex. It came out in therapy that her mother had told her that "men only want women for one thing." Her only way to fight her husband's criticism was by denying him "the only thing men want." She decided to become more assertive and to express her feelings verbally. Terror-struck, she defied him, and, to her amazement, he took the quiet role. After many arguments, she was able to explain to him how he was partially responsible for her condition. They both came for therapy, and as the criticism and anger diminished, her weight followed and went down. Their sexual activities, while not yet perfect, are more pleasurable and frequent. Sex has become a bond instead of a weapon of mutual abuse.

Lynn was a normal, sexually active, young divorced woman. While her marriage had been unhappy, her relationships after her divorce were pleasant. She had met a man, fallen in love, and planned marriage. Three months before the wedding date, he suddenly informed her, in a letter, that not only was he running off with another woman, but he was using some of Lynn's savings for the down payment on a home in another state! Stunned, she began to gain weight. As her opportunities for sex decreased, she retreated into a fantasy world of masturbation and sexual devices. She was now a sharply critical person and eighty pounds overweight. The less attractive she got, the more she withdrew, until her life centered on food. She was hospitalized and given psychiatric treatment.

At first, her motivation to change was low, because she had retreated so fully into the fantasy world. After a while, we enlisted the aid of close friends to help restore Lynn's confidence. Now she has lost weight, is dating cautiously, and has attempted sex. She still won't allow herself to feel any emotion for her partners. Restoration of her normal weight is a factor vital to her future happiness.

Bob was grossly obese and in his late thirties. He was found upon examination to have glucose intolerance and insulin insensitivity. He had little desire for sex, and his overeating was already a substitute for the lack of companionship. He often fantasized about reducing, but was either unable or unwilling to do so. When he did want sex, it was hard to find partners willing to experiment with the limited positions available to an obese person. He developed inferiority feelings and ate more. After being placed in psychotherapy and on a reducing regimen, he lost 80 pounds in 6 months. At that time he started to feel sexual stirrings. After losing 50 more pounds, he had a sexual encounter. Sex and weight loss encouraged each other, until he has now lost 144 pounds (65 to go!); his self-esteem has improved, and his blood sugar and metabolism are normal. There certainly was a definite relationship between sex and obesity in Bob's case.

At this point, I would like to make some observations about the psychological causes of obesity. Like stress smokers and drinkers, heavy eaters are often driven by stress of some sort. Depression and its underlying hostility can also contribute. Resentment against working conditions, employers, the system, or relatives can lead to face-stuffing. A wife can resent her husband's work because it takes him from her. Nagging and lecturing loved ones on thinness can drive them to food. And, finally, Richard Stuart said, "Obesity can be a modern chastity belt." I believe it can also be used as a cudgel to get even with a spouse.

The Pregnant Father Syndrome

Becoming parents often affects the eating habits and weight of both the mother and father. There are many reasons why a pregnant woman eats. She can feel that she is being robbed of essential nutrients, or that the baby is parasitically draining her health. She can feel the pressures of losing her figure, losing her husband's attention, having new duties, not looking good, being advised to curtail sex, or being blamed for an unwanted pregnancy. After the baby is born, she has no free time; she must share the husband's attention with the baby; and, most important, she often has an overly romantic ideal of marriage, beside which the real thing is disappointing. All of these problems can precipitate overeating.

The young "pregnant father" is not immune to stress. He often is reluctant to admit that he wanted the child. He can be afraid of the financial responsibilities of parenthood. He too has lost freedom and must share duties around the house. Startlingly, we have found among our patients an average weight gain of thirty-seven pounds as these men ate away their feelings of resentment and jealousy! These husbands need counseling and diets, or else after the birth of the baby they may continue their bad eating habits. We have seen "pregnant fathers" either demanding sex or withdrawing from it after the baby arrives—especially if the mother is too devoted to the child. The sex so demanded is more frequent but often less tender and fulfilling than usual.

Barbara, a teenager, had problems of a different sort. She was a plain-looking girl, not popular at school, with a beautiful sister. Barbara's mother would harass her about getting dates and tell her she might never get a husband. Barbara's grades, better than those of her popular sister, suffered because of the nagging, and Barbara started to eat. Feeling too much was expected of her, she used food as an escape. She would go on dates that her sister got for her, and she soon discovered sex. Afer she had established a reputation for being a "round heels" her sexual and eating habits stimulated each other until they were both way out of control. During psychotherapy she learned that this behavior was a rebellion against, and a punishment of, her mother for all her pressuring. Barbara felt that if she became fat enough, no one would want her, while if she was thin, she would have to attempt to be liked for herself—a scary thought. Finally, no one would ask her out, and her still-hyper sex urge went unfulfilled. Only then did she start to reduce. It has been two years, and she has lost weight, limited her sexual involvement to a steady boyfriend, and adjusted to a more normal life. There are still emotional scars, and her mother, with problems of her own, is indifferent to Barbara.

Loraine's overeating bordered on bulimia; her eating was almost sexual. Her moral standards prevented her from seeking a sexual outlet, and a severe depression resulted. Her tests showed diabetes, but she continued to stuff. She was given therapy and a diabetic diet. As she lost weight, the signs of diabetes diminished, and today she is on no insulin. Her sexual life is better, and she is engaged to be married.

Wilson, a hypoglycemic, is a similar case. His condition is complicated by the stress of coping with an unruly fifteen-year-old son he unwillingly got custody of in a divorce. The son's many legal, financial, and scholastic problems seem diabolically conceived to prevent his father's participation in a normal social or sexual life. In Wilson's case, the stress and related weight gain have continued to cause decreased sexual activity, frustration, and the physical symptoms of diabetes. He is still under psychiatric care.

When Mrs. X married, she had all the common ideas about a gallant gentleman on a white horse, singing romantic love songs written just for her. When these dreams were shattered, her mother-in-law suggested that the way to her husband's heart should be through his stomach. She cooked all of his favorite dishes, but he wasn't the type that gained weight. She, however, was! As she gained, he spent less and less time at home. Their sex life had been O.K., but as she became a mother-figure, his interest waned and he turned to extramarital affairs. She got fatter and fatter, until he had no more romantic feelings for her at all. When Mrs. X took her mother-in-law's suggestion to "lay down the law" to him, there was complete breach in their sexual relationship.

During therapy, we encouraged Mrs. X to get rid of the old bathrobe she wore around the house, pay more attention to her grooming, change her eating habits, and stop sitting around all day watching soap operas. Against our advice, she went on a starvation diet, and her weight yoyoed up and down. When we finally got her on a proper diet, with therapy and her husband's support, she was able to lose. At the husband's request, we brought his mother in and told her not to interfere any more. Mrs. X has gone from 235 pounds back to 143 pounds, and she and her husband share a normal pattern of daily activities. They have learned from the experience, and have used a negative problem to affect a positive change.

Sometimes oddball diets, exercises, pills, and even advice from the doctor don't deal with the causes of the overweight person's behavior. Treatment must seek to explore, examine, and explain the causes, and then encourage compliance to a sound plan to reestablish a normal, desirable type of behavior.

Millie had been sexually intimate with a young man. Later she met his brother, fell in love with him, and married him. Her new husband was unaware of the previous affair. She felt guilty and started to gain weight shortly after the marriage. During sex she sometimes visualized being with the brother, and this made her more guilty. Her 89-pound weight gain produced diabetic symptoms, even though she had no previous history of diabetes. She is currently under treatment for her emotional and physical problems.

We found that obesity leads to, or stems from, sexual difficulties in between 50 and 80 percent of the cases we have seen. A husband often blames his wife for weight gain. Her sexual desire may have increased, while his has decreased. This conflict leads to more eating on her part, more rejection—a vicious circle.

These problems can start in several ways: The man may never have satisfied his wife sexually; she may have a Victorian view of sex; she may experience no pleasure in sex; one partner may have a hormonal problem; or the woman may be in menopause and feel, mistakenly, that she is not supposed to want sex anymore. It is consideration and communication that will allow a couple to have sexual fulfillment and achieve weight loss.

We need to find the causes for obesity. What makes people eat? Are their sexual activities as good as ever? Has obesity limited the desire, pleasure, or frequency of sex? The purpose of sexual intercourse is to express love and experience pleasure. What happens is that obesity changes the desire. Often the woman's heightened desires cannot be met by the man whose lowered urges and distaste for his wife's appearance prevent a happy union.

Mr. A. has to prove that he is a big man in the boardroom, but often in the bedroom he is ineffective. At out-of-town conventions, he indulges in one-night stands to prove himself, but at home his performances are less than inspired. As he gets older, he yearns to recapture his youth. His wife has grown older too, and is less attractive, and heavy. Sooner or later there is rejection at home, which leads to more eating, more infidelities, and eventually to the ruining of the marriage. Many of these husbands want their wives to stay fat, because it gives the man an excuse to stray. We call this the "sabotaging spouse phenomenon."

Judy was the wife of a wealthy real-estate man and was 87 pounds overweight. She claimed that because she had been poor, she couldn't handle the temptation of her recent access to rich foods. Judy was pretty, but years of living "high on the hog" had increased her weight to 230 on a 5'5" frame. She knew nothing about nutrition and had to be taught about caloric values. Her concerned husband sent her to a private clinic to lose weight, telling her friends that she was in Europe. When she had attained her goal weight, her husband gave a big party in her honor and invited all of their friends to witness her "return from Europe." The guests were amazed at her beautiful figure, and her husband was proud of her. She got lots of compliments and offers to dance.

In the weeks following the party, she was invited for lunch dates, and soon her husband realized he was having to compete for her attention. His buddies were joking, "Better watch out, or someone will steal your wife from you!" The last straw came when he took her to get a new wardrobe, and the manager of the shop, an old boyfriend, was more than friendly. After the fitting, her husband took her to a restaurant, told her she looked haggard, and insisted that she eat a large meal. He then began to bring her candy and sweets and insist that she eat them.

She knew that she was doing wrong by eating the delicacies, but she wanted to please him, and he was very persuasive. When she gained weight back, he said that she looked better, but her friends were beginning to comment. She was torn between what she knew was right and what her husband seemed to want. When she came to us she complained:

> He is making me get fat, he hates to see me thin, but he does not like me to get the attention from other people. Even sexually I notice he is different. He makes demands on me sexually that leave me absolutely exhausted, and he continues to do this even more frequently than before, when our relationship was much more pleasant. His frequent demands for sexual activity are not only unpleasant to me, but I am unhappy about it because he is beginning to get violent about it. It is almost as if he is telling me—and he does tell me sometimes—"I'm going to satisfy you; I'm going to get you to the point of complete sexual saturation, and you won't even want anyone else, and you would not even want anybody else to even touch you." It's as though he is trying to drown me in sexual activity, which is really unpleasant and unsatisfying, and it is almost as though the violence of his sexual act is trying to make me unattractive to other people.

We had to call the husband in for psychotherapy, but the problem persisted and led to a divorce.

We found, in reviewing 4,000 obesity cases, that at least 50 percent of them had a sexual involvement, and 35 percent of those were of the sabotaging type. Sabotaging spouses tend to do three things: they tempt the dieter; they talk about how much they are enjoying *their* food; and they ridicule the fat person. These methods almost never help the dieter to lose. We feel that jealousy motivates these behaviors.

We had, in our clinic, a bookkeeper who was a poor sexual partner for his obese wife. He had always blamed it on her obesity. Finally she came in, took off 65 pounds, and became quite attractive. He, however, continued to have difficulty with sex. He tried to fatten her back up because his excuse was gone, but the problem persisted and led to divorce.

Preference for fat women can be another cause of diet sabotage. Some men like their wives fat, and if you dig into the man's background, you often find overweight mothers, fathers, or former lovers.

Sometimes just wanting company at the dinner table can cause sabotaging. In some families, mealtime is the only time the family spends together. The husband demands company at the table; the poor dieting wife sits there confronted with delicious, tempting food, and finally cannot resist. Sometimes, in these families, food is the only binding force. The wife may sabotage the husband, because if *he* loses weight, *she* may be expected to lose also. If she does, she feels that she won't be able to cook meals for the family and keep her nurturing-mom image. She's afraid of losing her family's love.

A wife's reducing can force a man to give up a pet activity, which he now justifies because of her fatness. He likes to stop off and have a few drinks with the boys. He really just wants free time, but he blames it on his fat wife, who is "always tired, and can't find a dress to go out in." A wife's fatness can remove the guilt of an extramarital affair. "I'm doing this because she's fat—it's her fault."

Some spouses associate a lean body with ill health and tell their mates that they are, or will be, unhealthy unless they gain. One wife worried her husband so much about a possible heart attack that he almost had one!

Often there are sexual side effects to the bypass and gastric stapling operations (two drastic weight-loss measures). In these, the stomach or intestines are blocked or removed to facilitate reducing. Weight losses of 37 to 55 percent are not uncommon. In some women an increased sexual desire has accompanied the weight loss.* The sex desire was so high in some, that hus-

* This may be due to the fact that stapling causes weight loss *in spite of* the high-fat, high-sugar foods being ingested.

74

bands were experiencing impotency, a fear of sex, and even the feelings that the wife was wanton and "not like the girl I married." One husband, who had been bisexual, became openly homosexual to avoid his wife's increased demands.

The rapid weight loss of a bypass operation can cause problems. One man, whose wife had ridiculed his poor sexual performance, came in for a bypass. As he lost, the ridicule decreased and sexual drive increased, but physical and psychological problems forced him to have the operation reversed. When he gained, the ridicule resumed. His wife finally pressured him to try stapling, and although he lost weight again, it wasn't slow enough for her. Her domineering is ruining the benefits of weight loss for him.

One husband's sex drive was so increased by a bypass operation, that his wife, formerly employed by him, had to seek work elsewhere to get away from incessant demands! I guess that it is safe to say that stapling or bypass operations are drastic, last-resort methods which can often *cause* as many problems as they cure. It is much safer to reduce in the normal way, if possible, because it gives the spouse time to adjust to the reducer's new image. The operations are sometimes necessary because the dieter is at the mercy of the spouse in a sabotaging relationship.

Tom was trying to lose weight. His wife was fat, and they had never had a good sexual relationship. Since he was a handsome fellow, his wife was secretly against his efforts to lose. She was afraid that if he reduced, she would have to do likewise, and she had many neurotic reasons for not wanting to. So she would sabotage his diet by putting butter in his food and refusing to give him what the nutritionist recommended. She increased her sexual demands, and he was unable to comply. Tom was diabetic and had high blood pressure. He needed desperately to lose weight, but she prevented it. In a final attempt to save his life, he shot and killed his

The intestinal bacteria could still be producing estrogens at an above-normal rate.—ADDANKI.

own wife and was sent to the penitentiary. He later died there of complications from his many health problems. We include this case to show how the various pressures of dieting are extreme and can lead to divorce and worse! We must be aware of the causes of non-nutritional eating: (1) a lack of sex, (2) boredom, (3) lack of affection, and (4) a need to prove oneself or punish others. We must decide if the obese person is afraid of his/her own sexuality, or has guilt feelings about it. He could either be punishing the spouse by denying sex or trying to prove that the spouse deserves nothing better than a fat, unattractive mate.

Bernadette Massey, a psychiatrist specializing in marital problems, has said that the divorce rate is as much as 84 percent higher in countries where dieting is popular. We feel that the problem is not the thin person, but the overweight one. Dieting can only be popular in countries where overeating is equally popular. Liz Taylor rationalizes that the thin, dieting wife, who is a bundle of nerves, will wreck any marriage. We disagree. Liz is not a psychiatrist. Women who are overweight are deluding themselves by seeing themselves as Liz Taylor-type sex objects. There is no glamour to a body swollen with fat.

Sometimes we do see a fat person being dated by an attractive, slim partner. This would seem to be a contradiction, but we have found that the normal-weight person with very strong feelings of inferiority feels comfortable only with a partner who is also inferior. The fat person *looks* inferior, and so there is equality.

You cannot change behavior unless you know what the behavior is. The attitudes behind weight gain go all the way back to feelings regarding sex, morals, and life itself. There are some guidelines we can follow when we are trying to help a dieter: Don't withhold sex, because it will add to the problem; don't discuss weight (or sex) publicly; don't nag or complain; and, finally, don't tease.

The starvation diet usually has a relationship with sex. Libido diminishes. At first, sex fantasies may occur, but after a while weight loss is the only thought. Prisoners of war often have these symptoms. In 1980, when the hostages returned from Iran, one of them had lost about forty pounds. When asked, "What is the first thing you are going to do you you get home?" he replied, "You mean the *second* thing!" (It was to sample his wife's cooking.) This humorous story illustrates the point that sex and hunger are basic, and our body signals tell us which one is more important at any given time.

When a person eats without hunger, it is often an attempt to patch up a bruised self-esteem, because your self-image is your greatest treasure. If we don't get self-respect, our sexual relationships are often the first things that suffer. Any time there is sexual frustration, there will be a replacement of that frustration by something else—drinking, eating, or extramarital affairs. The withdrawal of sex by a partner can lead to impotence, indifference, or infidelity.

In many cases, marriage stops at the dinner table. Meals are poorly prepared, and conversation is either tense or nonexistent. The compatibility of marriage is sacrificed on the altar of food. You cannot gain love or sex through food—only weight.

Diabetes and overweight are first cousins. Fernbarger says, "Treat the obesity before the diabetes; manage the obesity and you manage the diabetes." We can add, "Manage the obesity, and you often manage the sexual difficulties." There are sexual problems connected with all types of obesity, and with two-thirds of the twenty-six behavior patterns of obesity. Overweight is often the result of a central emotional problem of guilt, sex, possessiveness, greed, envy, jealousy, or security. Whenever these emotions are repressed, and can't be expressed in voluntary behavior, we have a type of chronic tension and a disturbance in health. The conflict causes more repression and eating disorders.

7

Diabetes and Sexual Awareness

S. V. Cherukuri, M.D., F.R.C.S. (Edinburgh),
Diplomat of the American Board of Urology

Diabetes is frequently associated with sexual dysfunction in males and females. The estimate of frequency of sexual dysfunction in men ranges from 40 to 60 percent. In females it is about 35 to 40 percent. The significance of these figures will become apparent when it is realized that there are at least 10 million diabetics in the United States.

Sexual Dysfunction and Impotency in Men

The impotency associated with diabetes can occur at any age. The published studies report a lower tendency for people in their twenties or thirties. About 25 percent of juvenile diabetics are impotent, whereas 50 to 70 percent of men over the age of 50 who have diabetes suffer this affliction.

Sexual dysfunction in men has many causes. For example, diabetic people are more prone to infection than nondiabetics. It seems that their white corpuscles are not effective in killing invading bacteria. Diabetic neuropathy (degenerative changes of the nervous system) can cause abnormal bladder function. This can lead to a serious infection which overpowers the white corpuscles and attacks the prostate. The prostate is a small gland between the bladder and the penis, which when infected, can cause painful and premature ejaculations. An infection like this can bring about a serious and prolonged lull in your libido.

Some diabetic men experience a diminished response to erotic stimuli. As time goes on, there may be a deterioration in the firmness or duration of erection. It is a sinister, slow process, which can take from 6 to 18 months. Sometimes the ability to ejaculate or experience orgasm remains, but it is the libido or interest which lessens. Do you find yourself buying *Playboy* for the articles? If so, your problem might be your diabetes, not your age, as was previously thought.

Several studies have been done on the hormonal status of diabetics. Testosterone, the male hormone, was found to be low in impotent diabetics by two separate researchers. W. Geisthovel found that "after a three-day stimulation with HCG the increase of basal total plasma testosterone was significantly lower in the two diabetic groups* in comparison with the normal person's." Berchtold et al., working in Germany, stated that "serum testosterone was markedly lower in diabetics than in normals." So the cause for the sexual problems in diabetic men can sometimes be due to the hormonal state, because the relative levels of testosterone regulate libido in men.

The impotency in diabetes can also be caused by diabetic neuropathy, a process of microscopic damage to the nerve tissue that occurs throughout the body. The exact cause for this neuropathy is not known, but a chemical substance called polyols, which produces segmental demyelination** and defective myelin synthesis,*** is deposited in the nerve fibers. This process is a result of hyperglycemia. The nerve fibers lose their ability to conduct stimulation from the brain to the penis, and erection is difficult or impossible.

* Impotent and nonimpotent.

** Segmental demyelination—destroy the myelin of the nerve tissue portion by portion.

*** Defective myelin synthesis—defective fat-like substance forming a sheath around narrow fibers.

Another problem can be changes or deposits in the small blood vessels to, from, and in the penis. This condition is called diabetic microangiopathy. The membrane of the blood vessels is thickened because of increased glucose content. This inhibits the flow of blood and again impairs erectile capacity. Larger blood vessels can be afflicted with arteriosclerotic lesions.

There is another type of impotence, known as "psychogenic impotence." This is the one where the doctor tells you that it's "all in your head." It is due to emotional problems; there are no organic problems associated with this type. Inability to achieve erection is, in this case, caused by psychological problems, just as in nondiabetic men. When diabetes is present, it is not the disease itself which caused this type of impotence, but the mental strain and worry associated with just having discovered that you have a serious and little-understood disease. To beat this type of sexual problem, it is necessary first to control other aspects of your life, such as the diabetes, your diet, your family life, and your job. Often when you normalize those things, your sexual problem will also improve.

Before you get too worried about psychogenic impotence, have tests performed to rule out the primary organic causes such as infections, diabetic neuropathy, or vascular damage. Doctors can now do this by monitoring nocturnal penile tumescence patterns. In this procedure, the male organ is observed during sleep. If erection occurs at this time, there is no organic basis for impotency. In 70 to 80 percent of such cases, sex therapy is likely to work. Vascular obstruction as a cause of impotency can be corrected by surgery.

A high percentage of obese men have potency problems. These are due primarily to the hormonal imbalance known to occur in obesity, but are further complicated by problems of low self-esteem and decreased attractiveness. In these cases, weight loss almost always improves the condition. Since obesity also leads to diabetes, there are two reasons to avoid it.

Impotency in marriage can cause numerous family quarrels. Some wives have been known to accuse their husbands of homosexuality or promiscuity. The ensuing discussions are often high in volume but low in communication. Health-care personnel coming in contact with diabetics should always take a sexual history to help the family understand *all* the possible problems associated with the disease.

Treatments

The sexual dysfunction due to infections in the prostate gland or the urinary tract can be corrected by antibiotic treatment from an appropriate physician. The diabetic neuropathy, or slow conduction by the nerve fibers, can sometimes be controlled by proper handling of diabetes. Once control is established, the nerve conduction is often improved and erectile capacity is restored. When major blood vessels are involved, this can be corrected by surgery. While this treatment is still in the experimental stage, the blood vessels to the penis can often be revascularized.

When there is complete loss of erection, due either to diabetic neuropathy or to small vessel involvement, a penile prosthesis can be implanted. The penile prostheses are of two types. One is a rigid type which causes permanent erection by the insertion of two silastic rods into the penile organ. During sexual arousal, the "glans" or head of the penis receives a generous blood supply, making the erection very satisfactory. The second device is an inflatable implant which is also surgically inserted into the penis. When there is sexual arousal, the implant can be filled with fluid, and erection will be maintained by a device in the scrotum.

I should mention a condition sometimes affecting diabetics called "retrograde ejaculation." In this condition, the seminal fluid flows backwards into the bladder at the time of orgasm, rather than coming forward through the distal urethra. This type of problem affects only about 1 or 2 percent of diabetics. It is due to autonomic neuropathy. Sufferers are infertile but enjoy otherwise normal sexual relations.

Sexual Dysfunction in Women

Until recently, the medical community ignored the complaints of sexual dysfunction in diabetic women. There were many publications in which it was mentioned that diabetic neuropathy does not affect women. However, in 1971 a survey was done comparing 125 sexually active diabetic women with 100 sexually active nondiabetic women—all between the ages of 18 and 42. It was found that 35 percent of the diabetic women reported being nonorgasmic in the preceding year. The other sexual disorder that is found in diabetic women is "dyspareunia," painful intercourse.

The reasons for the sexual disorders in the female are the increased incidence of vaginal and bladder infections due to increased sugar content in the vaginal mucosa. These patients are more prone to moniliasis infections (yeast infections). Bladder dysfunction due to diabetic neuropathy is common. The frequent bladder infections may also cause dyspareunia. The lack of orgasm is due to diabetic neuropathy. These woman need more stimulation, because of their increased threshold of sensory stimuli, to trigger the appropriate response. These diabetic women do not lose the capacity to be orgasmic, but they simply require higher levels of stimulus to set off the orgasmic reflex. The tragedy occurs when a couple, both diabetic, finds that the man cannot provide the sexual endurance and staying power needed by his wife. At the very time when she seems to need more stimulation, his ability is diminished. Unless the diabetic condition is diagnosed and reversed, the marriage, as well as the health of the partners, is in serious jeopardy. Occasionally, a couple being treated for diabetes will employ a vibrator to ease them through this trying time.

Sexual dysfunction in women can, of course, have

psychogenic causes. Common is the fear of the complications of pregnancy and the additional risks of congential defects in the children. Thoughts of these future problems prevent many diabetic women from enjoying a normal, spontaneous sex life. Fortunately, these fears can often be resolved by psychological counseling.

Several new approaches are necessary. Any time a patient, male or female, complains of sexual problems, undiagnosed diabetes must be suspected. Histories of diets followed and weights attained should be part of the routine questioning. Because diabetes is so closely related to diet, and normoglycemia so dependent on proper eating, a nutritional approach to sexual dysfunction practically suggests itself. Obesity, low self-esteem, diabetes, and impotency are all closely related.

8

Remission, Reversal, and Normalization of Adult-Onset Diabetes

In this chapter I will describe remission and reversal, or normalization, of diabetes. There are subtle differences in these terms you should know about.

Remission—the Unusual

Every doctor's dream is to be treating a chronic and hopeless disease and have it go away completely. In the history of diabetes there are a small number of cases where the patient, for one reason or another, enjoyed a complete disappearance of the symptoms.

Dr. Reed Harwood describes a twenty-four-year-old patient: "J.N. . . . was referred to my office with severe diabetes. He had . . . thirst, polyuria,* and weakness; his weight had dropped from 175 to 150 pounds. In recent months he had [been] drinking beer in considerable quantities and eating pretzels. During the next nine hours after admission he received 130 units of . . . insulin. [His] blood sugar fell to 53 mg./100 ml. He was discharged from the hospital two weeks later . . . on 80 units of lente insulin."

Dr. Harwood goes on to describe how J.N.'s blood sugar remained low for three months. Even though he had no hypoglycemic symptoms, his insulin dose was reduced to 50 units. He was on a 2,800-calorie diet of

---

* Frequent urination.

300 grams of carbohydrate, 130 grams of protein, and 120 grams of fat.

At the three-month point, he had a hypoglycemic attack. He was relieved with orange juice, and his insulin dose was lowered to 25. Three days later he had another attack, and insulin was stopped altogether. As long as he stuck to the diet, insulin was unnecessary.

A review of the literature of remission reveals a number of cases where diabetes has "disappeared" after various treatments. Naunym, an early researcher, said, "Diabetes mellitus may recover, but this happens very seldom, and I know of no case in which the cure of the disease has occurred after any long duration." F. M. Allen, realizing the need to distinguish between improvement and cure of diabetes, wrote: "A cured diabetic is one who can go and live like other people on the ordinary quantities of starch and sugar and remain permanently free from his former disease. . . . By such a test numerous cures are ruled out."

Recently, Newburgh and Conn reported that diabetes can "disappear" in obese persons who reduce, and that they not only remain sugar-free, but also regain normal glucose curves. Some who regain the weight reacquire the disease. Newburgh also reported that some of his diabetic patients remained diabetic in spite of losing weight. I feel that high-fat diet was probably responsible for these apparently conflicting cases.

Often when persons die of acute diabetes, autopsies are done to determine the effect of the disease on the pancreas. Interestingly, the pancreas in these cases seems to have undergone a constant struggle to regenerate those portions damaged by chronic overwork. It is now well established that the pancreas, unlike the brain, is able to repair itself after injury. In the case of a diabetic expectant mother, the child later showed excessive growth and production of the pancreatic islets. During the last months of her pregnancy, the mother's insulin need diminished. The fetus's pancreas, after becoming developed, was reacting to the high sugar levels by expanding its insulin-secreting ability.

An autopsy of a diabetic nine-year-old boy who had been killed in an accident revealed that his pancreas islets had regenerated during the time that his insulin dose had improved from 90 to 30.

The statistics show that in maturity-onset diabetes, marked remissions can occur quite often with prolonged dietary restriction and weight reduction. Juvenile cases of remission are rarer and seem to depend on early detection and vigorous insulin treatment, which keeps the blood-sugar level slightly low and gives the pancreas a chance to regenerate itself. The reason these cases aren't commonplace is that after a diagnosis of severe diabetes is made, and insulin is started, the natural tendency is to give just enough insulin to control hyperglycemia. Hypoglycemic attacks are feared, and every attempt is made to avoid them. It is much more likely that the patient prefers food to injections and so never gets his/her sugar level low enough to facilitate pancreatic rejuvenation. Even when remission occurs, relapses can be brought on by emotional upset, acute infections, or a poorly timed piece of pie.

The phrase "Once a diabetic, always a diabetic" is generally still true. Cases of remission where the person can resume a totally normal eating pattern are extremely rare, but those who are willing to follow a sensible diet can often remain symptom-free for the rest of their lives.

Reversal

Reversal or normalization of diabetic symptoms is a more realistic goal for adult-onset diabetics. While relatively few treated diabetics can return to their high-calorie, high-fat, high-sugar eating habits, most can become symptom-free by following a few easily implemented guidelines.

The treatment of diabetes through nutrition dates back to the late eighteenth century, when Rollo prescribed lime water, blood-and-suet pudding, and rancid meats, among other culinary delights. His advice never attained popularity.

H. P. Himsworth, as far back as 1935, discovered that diabetics, prior to their diagnosis, chose diets higher in calories, protein, carbohydrate, and particularly fat than did nondiabetics. High fat diets, he found, caused glucose tolerance impairment and insulin insensitivity. He also noted that the international variation in diabetics correlated with fat consumption.

West and Kalbfleisch found that in twelve different international populations, diabetes correlated positively with fat consumption, sugar consumption, and obesity. Diabetes was negatively correlated with complex carbohydrate consumption. The correlation with obesity was the highest (r equals 0.89), suggesting that overnutrition was the major problem.

Brunzell et al., in 1974 demonstrated that even diabetics using insulin or oral hypoglycemic agents experienced improved glucose tolerance on a high-carbohydrate, fat-restricted diet. Mann comments: "The mechanism for the decrease in fasting glucose levels during administration of the high-carbohydrate diet has been postulated as an increased insulin sensitivity."

So reversal or normalization becomes a matter of correcting the things which brought on the disease in the first place. We know now that these causal factors are high fat consumption, high simple sugar consumption, low fiber consumption, and overnutrition.

High fat consumption is easily corrected. Fat resides in most meats, oils, cream, butter, whole milk, and cheese. Start by substituting other foods for these, one at a time, and you'll soon notice improvement in your condition. Buy skimmed milk instead of whole. Reduce meat consumption by eating seafood, skinned poultry, or meat analogs several times a week. Buy the leanest cuts of meat. Substitute safflower or sunflower oil for lard, and margarine for butter. That will give you less saturated fat. If you can eliminate all pork, so much the better.

Inder Singh, working in India in the 1950s, was aware of the relationship between fat consumption and diabetes. Eighty patients with insulin-sensitive diabetes were treated with low-fat diets. Fifty became sugar-free in 3 to 6 weeks, 18 in 18 weeks, and needed no more insulin. Six still needed 10 units of insulin daily, and 6 more reduced their needs from 80–120 to 20–40. In describing his findings, I quote him liberally:

> Fat depresses the insulin mechanism. . . . If fat is reduced still further to the minimum, insulin begins to exert its curative effect, most patients can be stabilized on diet alone, and some patients are, to all intents and purposes, cured. Apparently when a diet low in fat is given, the diabetogenic stimulus is minimized, and insulin in adequate amounts can then cure diabetes. . . . Case 31 agreed to undergo estrogen therapy in spite of the risks, and was given 25 mg. of stilbestrol on alternate days for three weeks. He became considerably worse, and estrogen had to be stopped. He was retreated with diet and insulin for four weeks before he could be restored to the original state.

It is certainly frustrating to find that the basic mechanism of reversal of diabetes was known in 1935, proved again in 1955 and many times since, but still not accepted by the medical establishment in 1981.

Simple sugars, the mono and disaccharides, are what we call "sweets." All diabetics know that these are taboo, but often think that honey, brown sugar, molasses, or fructose are somehow better. They are all sugar, and even though honey and other fructoses are processed differently by the body, they can still cause hyperglycemic attacks. For dessert, eat fruits. You will be amazed how sweet raisins, oranges, and bananas taste when you haven't eaten sugar for a month or so. If you must sweeten your beverages, moderate amounts of artificial sweetener are much less harmful to the diabetic than sugar.

Overnutrition, the scientists' word for eating too much, is also easy to correct—in theory. In previous chapters I have tried to explain why weight loss is so difficult to achieve. I talked about nonnutritional eating, family and work pressures, and long-established habits. The diabetic can have a much easier time losing weight than the healthy person. The reason?—much stronger motivation. The overweight but otherwise healthy person has only one reason to lose weight—vanity. Usually this vanity is smothered by numerous countermotivations to eat—low self-esteem, love for food, fear of popularity, and the like.

On the other hand, you, the maturity-onset diabetic, have not only your pride in your appearance to motivate you, but the desire to become free of all diabetic symptoms, complications, and future problems.

Learn about calories. Keep track, mentally or on paper, of the number of calories you need to maintain an even weight. When you have established that, limit your daily intake by 600 calories. Since, for every 4,000 calories less than you need, you lose one pound, you will lose about a pound a week. Some of you will lose faster than others; don't get discouraged. There will be plateaus or times when you don't seem to lose at all. What is happening is that your body, used to more food, is adapting to the new amount. Your metabolism is evening out and learning to burn fat instead of storing it.

Eat breakfast, lunch, and dinner. You will feel better all day. Eat no simple sugars for the first month—especially at breakfast. Eat no more than two hundred calories after six in the evening. It's O.K. to eat two slices of whole-wheat bread before bed. If you eat more, not only will you not be hungry in the morning, but your sleeping body will store the rest as fat during the night. What else can it do? It only needs about twenty to twenty-five calories an hour to sleep. Refer to Chapter 15 frequently as a guide. Remember that, difficult as dieting is at times, it is always preferable to the alternative. I've done it, and so can you!

Fiber and Complex Carbohydrate

Fiber is simultaneously extremely important and widely misunderstood. An acquaintance of mine thinks that high-fiber foods—or "roughage," as he calls them—are foods which, like the sharp steel blades of a drainpipe-cleaning machine, scrape through the intestines, removing several layers of tissue along with the contents. He wants no part of them.

On the contrary, high-fiber foods are highly beneficial and do nothing but good in your system.* The most exciting work on this subject has been carried out, in totally separate studies, by James W. Anderson et al., John D. Brunzell et al., David, J. A. Jenkins et al., and others.

So much work has now been done on fiber and complex carbohydrate treatment of diabetes that it would fill a book by itself, and even this research is in its early stages. Since most fiber is not digested, nutritionists assumed that it was unimportant. I cannot tell the story any better than the research itself, and so I will briefly review the various papers on this exciting subject.

James Anderson, working in Kentucky, has researched the relation of fiber to diabetes; high-carbohydrate diets to diabetes; high-carbohydrate, high-fiber diets (HCF) to lipid metabolism; and the vitamin and mineral status on HCF diets. He concludes the following:

1. Diabetics can lower their insulin requirements on HCF diets; some could discontinue insulin.

2. HCF diets led to improvement in blood-sugar levels.

3. These diets lowered the blood cholesterol and triglyceride levels.

4. HCF diets reduce the likelihood of diabetic complications and hardening of the arteries.

* Some researchers have found that over the initial few weeks of a high-fiber diet, some minerals may be lost, but eventually the body adapts and corrects the problem.

5. Persons on HCF diets displayed no evidence of vitamin or mineral deficiencies for periods of up to four years (the length of the study).

Other researchers, working separately, have found the same thing. Brunzell, in Washington State, found that a high-carbohydrate (fiber) diet increased the sensitivity of the peripheral tissues to insulin. Hugh Trowell states that "high-fiber, high-carbohydrate diets caused remission of diabetes mellitus in many men who had been treated previously by oral agents or moderate doses of insulin. . . ." Jenkins reports that, "gelforming, unabsorbable carbohydrate* may therefore be a useful adjunct to anti-diabetic therapy, irrespective of the type of treatment or insulin dosage used."

In 1981, Simpson et al., summarized: "A diet high in complex carbohydrate and leguminous** fiber improves all aspects of diabetic control, and *continued use of low-carbohydrate diet no longer appears justified*". Miranda et al., from Chicago state that, ". . . increasing dietary fiber may be a useful means of lowering plasma glucose in some diabetic patients."

What is fiber? There are several kinds, according to T. J. Goulder et al. They define fiber as "the plant polysaccharides and lignin which are resistant to hydrolysis by the digestive system." They list the four major constituents as cellulose, hemicellulose, pectin, and lignin. Cellulose is found in all plants. It is not digested except by gut bacteria. Hemicellulose is found in many young plants, and while much of it is broken down in the colon, it is not absorbed by the body. Pectins are also found in young plants—mainly citrus fruits. Other fibrous materials include gums, gels, and mucilages, which are actually unabsorbable carbohydrates but not strictly fibers. Goulder notes that the latter are used in some explosives and thus gives fair warning to those of us including them in our diets for the first time. Go easy.

* Guar gum.
** Bean.

He also comments that "the mechanism of the diminished insulin response in . . . mild diabetics . . . may involve gut hormones as well. . . . Attainment of normoglycemia," he states, "is a major aim in the therapy of diabetes." I agree that this is feasible through high-fiber diets.

Fiber and Blood Fats

Anderson has studied the effect of various plant fibers on carbohydrate and lipid metabolism. He explains that celluloses bind water in the intestines. Lignins can bind bile salts and other organic materials. Hemicelluloses bind water and perform other physiological actions. Pectins form gels and bind water and bile acids.

He indicates that certain plant fibers,* when added to the diet, can reduce serum cholesterol concentrations. These are equally effective in animals and in humans. Triglyceride metabolism has been improved and reversals of hypertriglyceridemia have been reported in persons on high-fiber diets. Anderson concludes that high-fiber diets are accompanied by reductions in serum cholesterol values, short-term after-meal triglyceride values, and long-term fasting triglyceride values.

Other researchers have anticipated or corroborated Anderson's findings. Antonis pointed out back in 1961 that blood-fat values were lower in Bantu Africans who ate a high-fiber diet than in whites living in Africa and eating a high-fat diet (40 percent of calories). Groen found lower fat levels in Trappist monks than in Benedictines. Trappists eat less dietary fat than Benedictines. Scrimshaw said that "as the quantity of complex carbohydrate in the diet decreases, concentrations of serum cholesterol and especially triglycerides tend to rise." Shaper found a big difference in serum cholesterol and heart disease between Africans and Asians in

* Especially pectin, guar gum, and soluble fibers (gums, mucilages, and storage polysaccharides).

Uganda. Diet was the only major reason for this difference.

Since atherosclerosis is the most common cause of death in diabetes, it is doubly important to include a generous amount of various fibers in your daily diet.

Renewed Sexual Awareness—Men

Recent studies have shown that weight loss causes a 2½-fold reduction in androstenedione (estrogen raw material) and an increase in testosterone. With weight loss, the abnormal hormonal state normalized. Also, less fat tissue means less estrogen.

Gherman et al. believe that "in obese patients, severe caloric restriction rapidly corrects the SHBG* abnormalities similar, perhaps, to the rapid correction of insulin receptor abnormalities observed during starvation." What this means is that one of the main controllers of hormones, SHBG, is increased to the point where men retain their male hormone and excrete or get rid of excess female hormone.

Remember the Zucker "fat rats" that are genetically obese, with not only larger fat cells but more fat cells? They are also reproductively inadequate. However, Hemmes et al. showed in 1978 that "a high dose of testosterone . . . increases dramatically the litter production of young genetically obese male Zucker rats." They continue: "The reproductive inadequacy of the genetically obese male rat may be due to a deficiency of circulating testosterone." We have seen that obesity decreases testosterone in man in proportion to the degree of overweight. Losing weight reverses the testosterone loss and restores normal sexual libido.

Renewed Sexual Awareness—Women

In obese women, weight loss and dietary fat reduction bring similar benefits. The free, unbound testosterone

---

* Sex-hormone-binding globulin.

in their systems, caused by the lower amounts of sex-steroid-binding-globulin (SSBG), can cause menstrual irregularities, unusual ovulatory cycles, and unwanted body hair. Weight loss normalizes these problems and also helps regulate the unusually heightened sexual desire often found (and often unfulfilled) in these persons.

Post-menopausal women are popular subjects for sex hormone studies because their estrogen production is primarily extraglandular (outside of the glands). In one study, O'Dea looked at various hormonal levels before and during a fast-induced weight loss in obese post-menopausal women. He found concentrations of freely circulating testosterone (active) and estrogens increased in the obese women. After weight loss, the amounts of SSBG were normalized, and a drop in total serum estradiol and free testosterone occurred.

The bottom line is: *Most cases of adult diabetes are totally reversible through diet.* You won't be able to return to the eating habits that made you sick in the first place, but you will be able to lead a normal life. It took me sixteen years of constant research to discover and confirm that Western eating habits cause diabetes. I hope that I have saved you some time.

It won't be easy to change your eating habits, but for me, knowing *why* I should change gave me the needed motivation. I hope it does the same for you!

9

Obesity, Diabetes, and Cancer

How does nutrition relate to cancer? Experimenters have found three ways: (1) food additives or contaminants cause or help cause cancer; (2) deficiencies may weaken the body's defenses against cancer; and (3) changes in eating can cause metabolic abnormalities which increase the risk for cancer. We should not be hasty in blaming cancer on the action of a single cause or element. The relationship between nutrition and cancer is complex, and specific factors play only minor roles. It should be remembered that statistical correlation does not prove that one thing causes another. However, making a change in even one causative factor may be enough to prevent or reduce the chances of getting an illness.

Diet has been suggested as the major factor in the promotion of several types of cancer. In this chapter I would like to discuss the relationship of nutrition and obesity to cancer of the colon, breast, uterus, and prostate. Later I'll talk about food supplements and make some recommendations for lowering the risk of these cancers.

Two out of every seven persons get cancer; after age fifty, one out of three gets it. The reason it is important to learn what causes cancer is that the orthodox cancer treatments are so dangerous. If, in your lifetime, you get cancer, your physician will probably recommend one of the three types of cancer treatments: surgery, irradiation, or chemotherapy. All of these, in turn, either cause cancer or may cause it to spread.

In a way, we can't blame the physicians. Only a small minority of medical schools teach nutrition. I would like to suggest that we do everything we possibly can to keep from getting cancer in the first place. Cancer, like diabetes, is a degenerative disease spawned by our careless lifestyle. It doesn't attack us; we *encourage* it!

There are two theories about how carcinogens cause cancer: (1) the "one wrong molecule" theory, and (2) the "dose-related" theory. The first states that even one molecule of a cancer-producing agent can, if it enters your body, cause cancer. The second says that whether you get cancer is related to the amount of a carcinogen which enters your system. Because the average person consumes about five pounds of toxic substances yearly, I tend to feel that whether a given substance causes cancer in an individual is related to the dose. I also feel that a healthy human body, protected by proper nutrition, can fight off these agents. The problem occurs when a run-down body gets too big a dose of a cancer-causing substance. The first type of cancer we'll look at accounts for more new cases per year than any other type.

Cancer of the Large Bowel

North America, New Zealand, and Western Europe are areas of high incidence for cancer of the large bowel (colon). Africa, Asia, and Latin America don't have much of this type of cancer. Studies show that higher economic classes have more colon cancer and that it is strongly related to diet. Seventh Day Adventists have only 60 percent of the risk of bowel cancer that other Californians have, for instance. They eat much less dietary fat than other religious groups. Not only does dietary fat consumption correlate with colon cancer, but it strongly influences the metabolic activity of the intestinal microflora. I feel that this is the reason that people who eat a high-fiber diet avoid colon cancer. The slow transit time in the colon caused by a high-fat diet could allow bacteria to degrade intraluminal components, forming cancer-causing agents. Increased stool bulk could dilute these agents and render them less harmful.

A diet of high total fat and low fiber determines the concentration of acid and neutral sterol substrates (building blocks) in the colon, and the composition of the bacteria. The bacteria change these sterols into cancer-causing substances. Eight percent of colon cancer cases have elevated bile acid levels.

When two things are correlated, it does not prove cause, but if experimental evidence supports the correlation and the underlying causes can be described, the causal relationship is more likely. It has been established in the literature that there is a worldwide correlation between total fat consumption and incidence of colon cancer. We are concerned with the search for two things: cancer-*causing* agents, and cancer-*promoting* agents. There are so many types of fecal bacteria that trying to study individual types is a waste of time. It is more important to look at how different bacteria act than to identify them. Also it is interesting to see how diet affects the bacteria.

Reddy and Wynder found an increase in excretion of total bile acids in Americans consuming a high-fat, mixed Western diet, compared to groups not on such a diet. They concluded that the fecal bacteria of persons on a high-fat diet are more active in hydrolyzing many tumorigenic substances.

Experimental studies have verified the relationship between a high-fat diet and colon cancer. Rats were fed different amounts of fat and then given a drug known to cause cancer in them. The higher the fat content, the more tumors they got. Their colonic bile acid content was also elevated in proportion to the amount of fat in the diet. It seems logical that these changes in the metabolic activity of the microflora could alter the activity, toxicity, excretion, and reabsorption of cancer-causing substances. In other studies, different fibers, when in-

97

troduced into the diet, affected the circulation of bile salts to and from the liver, possessed various binding properties, and exerted a solventlike effect by diluting the cancer-causing compounds.

In another study, rats were again fed a high-fat diet, but were also given cellulose (a fiber). The group getting the fiber had fewer tumors, and fewer rats got tumors. Now, rats are not men, but . . .

On the basis of the study of cancer in different countries, in migrating populations, in persons who eat various types of food, and in animal models given cancer in the laboratory, we have seen an overwhelming amount of evidence pointing to dietary fat as a potent promoter of cancer. Later in the chapter I will discuss preventive measures.

Cancer of the Breast

North America and Western Europe are also high-risk areas for breast cancer. Asia and Japan are low in risk. Just this pattern alone makes one suspicious. When you see different rates in different countries, some envionmental factor is at work. In the West, the incidence increases after menopause, while in Japan the incidence remains unchanged during those years. Whatever causes breast cancer stays active after menopause in the West. (Readers with elephant memories will recall that estrogen production continues after menopause when you eat a high-fat diet.)

Western women living in Japan had the same incidence of breast cancer as other Japanese. When some of them moved to the United States, nothing happened for about two generations. But after that, descendants of these women had the same rates as American women! —more strong evidence for environmental factors. Polish immigrants changed their rates even faster, possibly because they fit into our society more quickly. Changes in diet appear to be the factor that best accounts for the increased risk of breast cancer experienced by migrating people.

A number of researchers have found a correlation between breast cancer mortality and daily consumption of fat. Animal fat seemed to correlate better than vegetable fat. The highest correlation was between cancer and pork consumption—followed by animal fat in general. The fat consumption in the United States had increased from 125 grams per day in 1909 to 156 grams per day in 1972. During that time deaths from breast cancer increased in the same way. Also, one need not be obese to get breast cancer; high-fat diet alone is enough to increase the risk significantly. In Japan, fat intake was 23 grams per day in 1957, and breast cancer deaths were about 1,600 for the year. In 1973, fat intake was up to 52 grams per day, and there were about 3,200 deaths that year. Even high-fat diet among *husbands* correlates with breast cancer in their wives!

To make sure that fat was the culprit, protein and carbohydrate content was held constant while the quantity of fat in the diet of rats was varied in several studies. The researchers found out four facts of interest: (1) the quantity of fat, independent of protein and carbohydrate, influenced the development of breast cancer; (2) the age at which the diet was started changed the results; (3) the reproductive history of the animals was important; and (4) calorie restriction had an effect.

The relationship of obesity to breast cancer has been reviewed. Obese mice have more mammary cancer than normal-sized ones. The high-fat effect is, however, separate from the high-calorie effect. A high-fat diet seems to promote rather than initiate cancer. We've all heard that in cancer studies huge amounts of the substances being studied are given to the subjects. In one experiment this was done on purpose. As the dose of carcinogen was increased, the effect of dietary fat *de*creased. This is important in the study of human cancer because the doses of toxic substances we are subjected to are very small. In our case, the effect of diet could be quite large—the reverse of the experimental situation.

To summarize the experimental studies, here are the

five important things we have learned: (1) dietary fat promotes, rather than initiates, breast cancer; (2) when the dose of carcinogen is low, the effect of promoting agents (diet) is high; (3) total quantity of fat is the central factor; (4) a certain amount of fatty acids is necessary to the high-fat effect; and (5) above a certain percentage, the amount of fat is not important.

How does a high-fat diet cause breast cancer? Steroids such as estrogen have been implicated in breast cancer. Prolactin, another hormone, has also been shown to be carcinogenic. Bandaru Reddy states that "the discovery of hypothalamic neurotransmitters capable of regulating prolactin secretion by the anterior pituitary led to the concept that circulating prolactin concentrations may be regulated by environmental factors acting on the central nervous system." Remember in a previous chapter when we talked about the "birds" sitting on the antennae of your brain's TV sets? The same thing happens here. Prolactin and growth hormone (a fat controller) are similar, so it seems likely that prolactin plays a role in fat metabolism. When you eat a high-fat diet, estrogens are produced. It has been demonstrated that drugs which antagonize estrogen action and block prolactin secretion retard tumor growth. I think that estrogens influence prolactin secretion and mammary tumor development. In rat breast cancer, the relative proportions of prolactin and estrogen are most important. Bandaru Reddy says, "Estrogens synthesized by peripheral aromatization of androgens could influence prolactin secretion patterns and, thereby, indirectly influence mammary tumor development." In plain English, more fat—more estrogen—more prolactin—more cancer.

Cancer of the Uterus

I would like to mention some of the factors associated with endometrial (uterine) cancer, and then try to relate them to diet. Higher risk for cancer of the uterus is connected with: (1) nulliparity (remaining childless), especially at younger ages; (2) early menarche, late menopause; (3) lower socioeconomic class (monthly rental as indication of class); (4) increased weight; (5) previous diagnosis of diabetes and hypertension; and (6) place of birth in North America or Europe. Obesity and breast cancer also correlate with cancer of the uterus. These facts, taken together, suggest possible connections with diet. Armstrong and Doll found that a high-fat diet correlated with uterine cancer as strongly as with breast cancer. Cole and Cramer postulated that dietary effects work through hormonal factors. Early menarche and late menopause would subject the body to prolonged estrogen insult. Obesity, previous diagnosis of diabetes, lower socioeconomic class, residence in North America or Europe, and breast cancer all are suggestive of high-fat, high-sugar, low-fiber diet. Obese tissue and intestinal microflora produce estrogens; these add to the hormones from the ovaries, adrenals, and placenta, and promote cancer.

Cancer of the Prostate

Prostate cancer seems to be another disorder caused by environmental factors. It occurs with some frequency among the elderly, but is not an important cause of premature death. Twice as many blacks as whites get prostate cancer. There are big international differences in the incidence of prostate cancer, strongly indicating that heredity is only a small factor. Various studies have shown a relationship with sexual drive and activity. These facts would suggest a hormonal connection. Armstrong and Doll found a strong correlation with dietary fat in their data about prostate cancer mortality. I think it's likely that the same factors are at play here as in other hormone-associated cancers. High estrogen levels in men are abnormal and could cause prostate cancer along with lowered sex drive. Prostate cancer is related to hormone secretion, retention, and target organ sensitivity. Any factor which affects these is suspect, and diet has a profound effect on hormonal systems.

101

Diabetes and Cancer

Bruno W. Volk and Klaus F. Wellman, in their paper entitled "Cancer and Diabetes," say that "the incidence of diabetes or impaired carbohydrate tolerance among persons with malignancies seems to be unquestionable." They review the literature and point out the correlations between diabetes and cancer.

Diabetic symptoms frequently accompany cancer and usually precede the cancer symptoms by about 2 to 6 years and precede the actual tumor by about 3 to 4 years. One study showed 63 hyperglycemics among 70 cancer patients. Another found that 52 percent of blood cancer patients had an abnormal glucose response, while only 8.5 percent of healthy control subjects had that type of response. In a study comparing malignant cancer patients with those with benign tumors, 36.7 percent of the first group had abnormal glucose tolerance, while only 9.3 percent of the second group did. Table 9.1 lists various types of cancer and shows the percentage of persons with abnormal glucose tolerance.

Table 9.1

Type of Cancer	Percent with Abnormal Glucose Tolerance
Uterus	64
Skin	47
Soft tissue	44
Floor of mouth	45.5
Lymphosarcoma	54.5
Hodgkin's Disease	50
Thyroid	70
Pancreas	80

Keep in mind that only 1 to 10 percent of any given population normally has diabetes. The relationship of diabetic symptoms to cancer is very complex; specific cause and effect connections are impossible to make at this time. However, certain commonsense observations are inescapable. We are exposed to numerous cancer-causing substances daily, but only some of us actually get cancer. It is safe to say that cancer, like diabetes, is largely a degenerative disease that we *allow* ourselves to get. Strong, healthy bodies fight off the many foreign substances ingested into our systems. Only when our immune systems are impaired do the toxic compounds get a foothold. We'll discuss preventive measures shortly, but it seems justified at this time to recommend what has been called by many a "prudent diet," involving reduced calories, fats, and sugars, and an increase in complex carbohydrates and fiber.

Increasing Your Defense Budget

In cancer research, a growing body of evidence is suggesting that a proper approach to cancer prevention and treatment is through nutrition. Since traditional medicine is oriented toward curing disease (and what a tremendous job it has done—infectious disease accounts for only 3 percent of total yearly deaths), the idea of prevention is new and in its fledgling stage. The most exciting thing about nutritional therapy is that it is so much safer and easier than orthodox cancer treatment. Many types of nutritional therapy have been tried, and the results are often better than traditional treatment, and never worse!

Ruth Long, Ph.D., in her series of booklets on nutrition and cancer, starts by emphasizing that good nutrition helps keep all the body's cells healthy. With proper nutrition, Ruth claims, we can not only keep from getting cancer, but actually reverse certain types. With various diets, tumors have been actually dissolved and passed from the body! She feels that traditional therapies sabotage the body's immune system and prevent it from fighting the tumor.

She has lists of foods that are either recommended, allowed in small quantities, or forbidden. In general she favors whole grains, fresh fruits, steamed vegetables, and salads. You are to limit your use of teas, legumes, butter, and water (you need stomach space for juices). You must avoid animal protein, alcohol, tobacco, drugs, dairy products, and refined or processed foods. Dr. Long suggests three main meals per day with three small snacks in between. She feels that supplements are needed to make sure you are getting all the nutrients necessary to protect your cells from cancer.

Several single nutrients are very important in the body's ability to fight misbehaving cells. Vitamin A has been proved to be able to prevent cancer of the mouth and respiratory tract. Cancer patients have been treated with anywhere from 5,000 to 25,000 I.U. of this vitamin with good results. The whole family of B vitamins is necessary for the efficient operation of the immune system. A property of vitamin C is its ability to prevent uncontrolled cell division. In a study of vitamin E and rat skin cancer, rats protected with vitamin E had much less cancer than the control group given corn oil instead.

Certain minerals are vital to cancer protection. Selenium, when present in the soil of a country, seems to protect the inhabitants from cancer. A certain type of mouse which develops spontaneous breast cancer at a rate of 82 percent was treated with selenium. The rate in treated mice was only 10 percent.

We can fight cancer in three ways: (1) reduce the number of carcinogens we are exposed to, (2) increase the number of anti-carcinogens we are exposed to, or (3) do both. We have much more control of the food we eat than anything else, so it is the best place to start. The high intake of fat in the diet, combined with deficiencies of vitamins A, B, C, E, and selenium may relate to the causes of several common cancers.

Recommendations

As I was writing this chapter, a report in the newspaper told of a new study linking pancreas cancer with coffee drinking. I mentioned it to a couple of friends, and one said. "Anyone can quit drinking coffee; it takes a real man to face future cancer." It is true that life presents us with hundreds of difficult decisions on a daily basis. In our youth many of us feel that nutrition is something we can correct later. In our quick-cure society, the disease comes before the treatment.

In cancer prevention, the reverse is often the case. It is imperative to educate our young people to the fact that the diseases they will someday face will have been caused largely by environmental factors—factors under their control. If you are a parent, start teaching your children about nutrition at an early age. I know how hard it is to wean them from sweets and junk food after they have gotten used to them. It would seem that a national effort might work better than an individual one, but with the big food-processing companies in the way of legislation, progress will be slow.

In the meantime, please follow this advice. Cut down on your consumption of these things: (1) fats—both animal and vegetable, (2) fried foods, (3) salt and pickled foods, (4) alcohol, (5) nitrates and nitrites, (6) refined carbohydrates. Increase your use of: (1) fresh fruits and vegetables, and (2) fruit, cereal and vegetable fiber.

Added to your food, you should take, as a preventive measure, supplements of the following elements: (1) vitamins A, C, E, and B; (2) a multimineral supplement; and (3) 50–150 micrograms of selenium and chromium. These nutrients will be your health-insurance policy for the future. I know that your physician may have told you that taking vitamin supplements is a waste of money because you "get all you need in your food." That was true when he was in medical school, but it is no longer the case. Because of the way modern farming and processing is done, the amount of nutrients in food has been drastically reduced. The supplements are a very cheap measure when compared to the cost of treating a terminally ill cancer patient (about $100,000). An ounce of prevention if you will.

Carlton Fredericks recommends the following daily amounts of supplements:

Table 9.2

Selenium	50–150 micrograms (mcg)
Vitamin E	400–1200 units
Vitamin A	5000–25000 units
Vitamin C	250–2500 milligrams (mg)
Vitamin B_6	10 mg
Inositol	500 mg
Choline	1000 mg
Vitamin B_1	5 mg
Vitamin B_2	5 mg
Niacin	50 mg
Vitamin B_{12}	25 mcg
Folic acid	100 mcg
Biotin	30 mcg
Pantothenic acid	100 mg
PABA	30 mg
Vitamin D	400 units
Bioflavinoids	25 mg
Iron	50 mg
Calcium	40 mg
Magnesium	7 mg
Manganese	6 mg
Copper	.25 mg
Zinc	.18 mg
Potassium	.1 mg
Betaine HCl	25 mg
Lysine HCl	10 mg

In regard to food additives, Adelle Davis's advice still provides a humorous rule of thumb: "If you can't pronounce it, don't eat it."

10

Hypoglycemia vs. Diabetes

Hypoglycemia is a widespread condition of temporary low blood-glucose level which affects about fifteen million Americans. Its frequent labeling as a nondisease has led to its being little understood. Actually, the term "hypoglycemia" encompasses a group of related disorders, so proper diagnosis is very important to choosing of a treatment.

The three main types of hypoglycemia are: fasting hypoglycemia, functional hypoglycemia, and exogenous (drug-induced) hypoglycemia. Fasting hypoglycemia is present before meals and upon waking. It is characterized by an overabundance of insulin action without the stimulus of food. During a fast, the blood-sugar level gets lower and lower. The pancreas produces insulin when none is needed. Fasting is poorly tolerated by the person with this disorder. Fasting hypoglycemia can be caused by cancer of the pancreas, liver disease, alcohol abuse, poor nutrition, or other glandular diseases. Drug-induced hypoglycemia is caused by an overdose of insulin or an oral hypoglycemia agent.

Functional hypoglycemia, the most important one to our subject, includes two distinct types: reactive-functional hypoglycemia, and functional secondary to early diabetes. Reactive hypoglycemia is associated with an immediate overresponse of the pancreas to a meal high in refined carbohydrates. An oral glucose-tolerance test shows no hypoglycemia before meals. After the carbohydrate load is given to the subject, the blood-sugar level rises slowly but never reaches diabetic levels. It then declines to below 50 milligrams per 100 milliliters between the second and fourth hour and then rebounds spontaneously. Symptoms are possible but not always present. Insulin release is prompt but excessive.

Functional hypoglycemia secondary to early diabetes is different from reactive hypoglycemia in that there is a delay between the administration of the glucose load and the release of insulin. There is an early hyperglycemic peak, often over 400 milligrams per 100 milliliters, which remains for one or two hours. Blood sugar then falls quickly to abnormally low levels.

If you throw an object at an angle only slightly above horizontal, it will follow a gently trajectory to the earth. If, on the other hand, you throw it at a seventy-five-degree angle from horizontal, the descent curve will be similarly steep. Fig Newton's law of glucose states that, in hypoglycemia, WHAT GOES UP COMES DOWN A GREATER DISTANCE. A meal containing refined carbohydrates causes the blood-sugar level to rise. When the oversensitive pancreas squirts insulin into the bloodstream, the level drops not just to normal levels but below normal. It is the steepness or speed of the fall which usually brings on the symptoms, not the low level itself. About 10 percent of the population have hypersensitive pancreases which respond this way.

Symptoms

In some, the effects are mild, bordering on humorous. Drowsiness, restlessness, lack of concentration, forgetfulness—all these symptoms can be passed off as minor goofiness. Aunt Flora, after a big dessert, wanders around the house looking for her glasses (they're on her head), the newspaper, a chair—struggling to make simple decisions and movements. She may not even know that her behavior is abnormal. Others who don't know of her condition think she is drunk or neurotic.

In others the symptoms can be more serious: irrational behavior, emotional instability, distorted judgment, nasty personality defects, dizziness, fainting or blackouts, fatigue or exhaustion, narcolepsy, muscle pains or cramps, cold hands and feet, numbness, insomnia, nightmares, irritability, crying spells, nervous breakdown, worry, anxiety, depression, illogical fears, suicidal thoughts, tremors, cold sweats, inner trembling, uncoordination, convulsion, fast or irregular heartbeat, blurred vision, allergies, itching and crawling sensations, neurodermatitis, arthritic pains, gastrointestinal upset, loss of appetite, loss of sex drive, impotency, dry or burning mouth, ringing in ears, temper tantrums, noise and light sensitivity, shortness of breath, peculiar breath or body odor, nausea, or hot flashes. Whew!

The sufferer is often considered a crank or complainer by his associates, a hypochondriac by his doctor, and a neurotic by everyone else.

Hypoglycemia and Drugs

Hypoglycemia can be aggravated by many over-the-counter and prescription drugs. The actions of anti-inflammatory drugs, analgesics, anticoagulants, antibiotics, diuretics, hormones, stimulants, tranquilizers, nicotine, caffeine, and alcohol can all have an effect on metabolism. The sugar in medicines is a problem for many. Malnutrition and abnormal liver and kidney functions can make hypoglycemia worse. Think about it. In the morning many people start the day with coffee, a sweet roll, and a cigarette—caffeine, sugar, nicotine. What a nutritious combination! And this is supposed to nourish your body until noon? You'll be lucky if that "meal" sustains you for two hours. Additional doses of the same "food" are then craved throughout the morning—adding to the low-blood-sugar problem. You pancreas is kicked around like a soccer ball and forced to spit out insulin like a fire hose gone wild.

It wouldn't be so bad if you ate this way only occasionally, but many of you follow this plan chronically. Is it any wonder that the morning traffic, the parking-lot attendant, your receptionist, secretary and boss all seem to be bent on harassing you? Give your body and brain something good to eat, and they will cooperate with you all day. The folks promoting good breakfasts are not just out to sell eggs. When you wake up, you haven't eaten for fourteen hours. (Unless you stuffed you mug before bed.) Why would you want to start each day of your life with three nonfoods?

Gum Control

Studies have been done lately which strongly link hypoglycemia and crime. One researcher discovered that the brain waves of persons with low blood sugar were abnormal. He noticed that starving the brain cells fogged the moral sense and distorted the conception of his subjects.

Children in particuliar are susceptible to food-related sociopathy. Dr. Joseph Wilder, a New York psychiatrist, found that in poorly fed children the growth of the brain can be retarded, altered, or stopped. He says: "The child may be neurotic, psychopathic, and be subject to anxiety, running away tendencies, aggressiveness, a blind urge to activity and destructiveness, with impairment of moral sensibilities. In its simplest form, it is a tendency to deny everything, contradict everything, refuse everything, at any price."

Hypoglycemia has been related to juvenile delinquency. A study of 129 delinquents determined that 116 of them had low blood sugar. Considering the many symptoms of this disorder, it would seem prudent at least to examine the diet of anyone, particularly a child, whose behavior is inappropriate and unexplained.

Suggestions

If you have any of the symptoms of hypoglycemia and don't know why, ask your physician to order a six-hour oral glucose-tolerance test to determine the possibility of hypoglycemia. It could be that the mental and physical complaints you have been putting up with could be easily reversed through proper nutrition. If so, avoid white sugar and flour. Eat less fat and more complex carbohydrates like grains and vegetables. Watch the sugar content of convenience foods, medicines, and sauces. Eat more fiber. Don't smoke tobacco or drink alcohol. If these recommendations sound familiar, you are getting the point. Treating hypoglycemia is no different from merely eating prudently. By repeating these guidelines, those of us who care about your health hope to make worldwide changes in eating behavior. When people realize that the prudent diet is not just some sadistic health nut's way of punishing others but the way to avoid many degenerative diseases, I'll be out of a job. In the meantime, I can't rest until I make the information available to all.

11

Alcohol—Dragster Fuel and Altered Sexual Awareness

QUESTION: What goes full speed for a short period of time and then rests for a long period?

ANSWER: A dragster or a drinker.

Alcohol is a perfect fuel for a drag racing car. These roaring, smoking monsters are created for one purpose only—to accelerate from a standing start to the end of a quarter-mile strip in as short a time as possible. Between races, the cars are torn down and all the parts that broke, wore out, or suffered stress are replaced, at high cost, by new ones. Dragsters are driven only a tiny fraction of the time; the rest is spent in their repair, refurbishment, and careful tuning to keep these fickle fast-starters running.

If this is the way you want your body to spend its time—working only a fraction of the time and being repaired the rest—alcohol would be a good choice of food for you. Most of us, however, prefer to have our bodies working all the time and needing repair only infrequently. For us, alcohol is much too fast-burning.

Alcohol and sugar are similiar foods in several ways. Like sugar, alcohol is almost a nonfood; it has calories but no nutrients. It is very fast-burning and raises the level of glucose, lipids, and triglycerides in the blood. As a food it is poor; as a drug, worse. Nathan Pritikin points out the bad effects of excessive alcohol. It: (1) causes liver damage, (2) reduces oxygen-carrying capacity of the blood, (3) depresses your immunity system, (4) complicates arthritis, (5) destroys judgment, (6) irritates urinary tract and prostate, (7) endangers pregnant women, and (8) disrupts family life.

If alcohol were just a poor food, no one would drink it, because its taste, in pure form, is anything but appetizing. The reason so many people drink it is because of its druglike properties. I know *you* don't drink it for that reason, but some people actually do. Really! Millions, in fact.

Why do some people become alcoholic? Cheraskin and Ringsdorf feel that improper nutrition can lead to alcohol abuse. They point out that the alcohol preference of laboratory rats can be influenced by the diet given to them. Three groups of rats were fed as follows: Group 1—high-sugar diet; Group 2—high-sugar diet plus supplements; Group 3—nutritious diet. All groups were offered water and a solution of 10 percent alcohol in water as beverages. Group 1 showed a strong preference for the alcohol solution. The rats in Group 2 showed no particular preference for either drink. Group 3 drank mostly water. When the booze-tippling members of Group 1 were switched to a nutritious diet, they went on the wagon. Conversely, when the well-fed, teetotaling Group 3 rats were put on the high-sugar diet, they developed a taste for the hard stuff.

Alcohol seems to be like sugar in another way. When taken into the body, it produces a later craving for more of the same. Since 70 to 90 percent of alcoholics have functional hypoglycemia (see Chapter 10), it seems likely that low blood sugar plays a big part in these cravings. Abnormal metabolism caused by poor diet, but aggravated by the use of alcohol (and nicotine and caffeine), could simmer for years before alcoholism begins. All these drugs are well known to cause strong psychological dependencies that are not easily broken.

Why don't alcoholics just stop? Because very few are willing to take the famous "first step"—that of admitting that they are weak-kneed about alcohol and that

113

their lives have become unmanageable. Alcoholics "decide" to start drinking, but only "wish" to stop. After years of alcohol abuse, they actually feel worse as they attempt to quit than they feel as alcoholics—much like a heroin addict during withdrawal.

Alcohol and Altered Sexual Awareness

Alcoholics actually suffer hormonal imbalance. Alcohol given to healthy men dampens testosterone secretion, decreases the blood content of this hormone, increases the rate of clearance of the male hormone from the body, and does all this independently of its ill effect on the liver or on nutrition. A team of scientists studying the feminization found in alcoholics discovered that estrogens, prolactin, neurophysin, and sex-steroid-binding gloubulin were all elevated twofold in their subjects. They concluded that the ratio of estrogens to prolactin could be a factor in the growing of breasts and other changes in secondary sex characteristics common in advanced alcoholic men. They also state that alcoholic men have an absolute increase in plasma estrogens. In cirrhosis of the liver, testosterone is changed to estradiol (E_2), while androstenedione (another male hormone) is changed to estrone (E_1). This estrogen production is also a cause of diabetes.

Alcohol impairs both the hypothalamic-pituitary and gonadal functions. When alcohol changes the blood content of lutinizing hormone (LH), primary gonadal failure and hypothalamic-pituitary suppression are the result. Remember the birds which, in Chapter 5, confused the signals that control insulin production? In the case of alcohol, the birds mess up the signals to the male's sex glands. More female hormone than male hormone is produced, and feminization occurs.

Kley et al. studied the binding to sex-hormone-binding hormone of sex steroids in men with fatty liver, hepatitis, and cirrhosis of the liver. In these subjects he found an increase in estrone, a smaller increase in estradiol, and an increase in LH. There was a drop in testosterone (T) in the men. The ratios of E_1 and E_2 to T were both elevated and were singled out as the probable cause of feminization. Chopra et al. found that male cirrhosis patients with female-type breast development had high ratios of estradiol/T.

Alcohol and Abnormal Carbohydrate Metabolism

Alcohol abuse causes the same type of metabolism problems that sugar use causes. When large amounts of alcohol enter the bloodstream quickly, the pancreas (especially the one in ten that is hypersensitive) is stimulated to produce lots of insulin. Not knowing when to quit, it continues this overproduction, much like an overzealous fireman dousing a smoker's match with a flood of water from his hose. When the fireman is done, the match (and smoker) is cold and soggy and the water supply is diminished unnecessarily. When the pancreas finally stops, your blood-sugar level is too low and your pancreas is strained by the effort. Misused in this way, the pancreas becomes more sensitive and starts overproducing insulin regularly, shortening its life (and yours) in the process.

Alcohol and Nutritional Deficiency

Since alcohol is so high in empty calories, it displaces other foods in our diet. For example, let's say that you need 2,500 calories a day to maintain your ideal weight. There are three ways that you can add 900 calories of alcohol to your diet (about four drinks). You could add the 900 calories to your present 2,500 and gain a pound of extra weight every 6 days. Or, to stay the same weight, you could subtract 900 calories of good food from your diet and replace them with the alcohol. What most drinkers do is replace *some* of their diet with alcohol and gain weight at a more moderate rate —several pounds a year. At your new amount of food, let's say 2,000 calories a day, it will be harder to squeeze all the necessary nutrients into each day's allotment. Deficiencies will develop and increase your chances of getting many nutrition-related diseases.

You be the judge. Alcohol abuse can cause liver dysfunction, nutrition deficiency, diabetes, hypoglycemia, low resistance to disease, poor judgment, feminization, impotency, hormone imbalance, bladder problems, birth defects, and an unhappy family life. Alcohol is a poor food for human beings and a powerful drug. Some of you might choose to be like the dragster—exciting the crowds on the weekend and recuperating in the repair shop Monday through Friday. Others have too many things to accomplish to be "down" 85 percent of the time. Which are you?

12

Overeaters Anonymous and Obesity

I wasn't quite sure what to expect as I pulled into the church parking lot to attend a meeting of Overeaters Anonymous (OA). I was greeted at the door by a friendly middle-aged woman and asked to sign my first name and telephone number. I took my place among a seated group of persons of all ages, mostly females. We were asked to join hands in a circle to open the meeting with a short prayer. As I fumbled to comply, my initial nervousness was partially comforted by the slight hand squeeze given to me by a friendly neighbor. After the prayer, a young woman, presumably the leader, got up in front of the group and read several passages from one of a selection of pamphlets lying on the table.

Then each person in turn was given the chance to read from another pamphlet. This reading was voluntary, and no one minded if someone did not wish to read. Following this, each person introduced himself or herself by first names, and included the fact that he/she was a "compulsive overeater." Each one could, but was not required to, talk about anything related to progress in the program. Topics ranged from having "abstained" just for that day to having attended a retreat sponsored by the group. The talk centered around "abstaining," "Higher Power," or self-esteem.

After the individual talks, a break was called, and some people helped themselves to low-calorie refreshments. As no formal invitation was extended, I did not partake. Following this, the main speaker was to address the group. I sat up to listen. Another member discussed his various dietary ups and downs. The meeting ended with another prayer, more hand squeezes, and a vocal exhortation for all to "keep coming back."

I admit that I was somewhat confused as I left this meeting about what had been accomplished. The question is difficult to answer after only one meeting, but some thoughts come to mind. Overeaters Anonymous is a long-lasting program through which individuals can make a permanent change in their behavior. It stresses that eliminating compulsive overeating is important in a member's life. In return for this help, members must invest a tremendous amount of themselves. Families are advised that the overeating member will be changing in many ways. There will be constant contact with a "sponsor," telephone calls at all times of the day, and meetings to attend. Unfamiliar behaviors and attitudes may perplex and annoy the family. Feelings that were up to now hidden will be coming out into the open. Success can be easy or difficult, quick or time-consuming. The family must cooperate.

To love others, a person must love himself. It is this self-esteem that OA attempts to restore to the individual. A twelve-step plan forms the basis of the method, and constant support from the group keeps members from straying away from the plan.

OA's goal is to help its members stop compulsive overeating by following a medically approved plan of eating, with the support of a sponsor. Beginning with the first meeting, it is followed one day at a time. Personal action and service to others are two important parts of the solution. A member is free to choose his sponsor, food plan, and definition of "Higher Power." Sponsors are other members who are currently abstaining. Several food plans are offered. Your "Higher Power" can be God, the group, your sponsor, or any other personal definition you want.

The food plans offered included: Basic Four, Sugar and Flour Free, Vegetarian, Youth, Medical, Modified Carbohydrate, No Refined Carbohydrates, and Maintenance. All diets contain about 30 percent fat and "sufficient" protein and carbohydrate. Refined carbohydrates are not recommended, while supplements are.

Recovery is hoped for on three levels: emotional, spiritual, and physical. On an emotional level you are helped to think about food as being needed to sustain life, not to face it. It should not be used to help you cope with feelings, nor for comfort or oblivion. On the spiritual level, you are encouraged to surrender your will power to your Higher Power—something outside yourself. Physically, you are to see overeating as a highly visible illness. You are encouraged to eat to live, not live to eat.

Several guidelines are offered to the recovering compulsive overeater. Three moderate meals per day are suggested, with no-cal or low-cal beverages in between. Refined starches, sweets, gluttony, meal-skipping, and second helpings are discouraged, while moderation, telephone calls to group members, and more communication in general are recommended.

The group concepts are unity, autonomy, and anonymity. The welfare of the group comes first. Each group is free and self-directing, except in matters which affect other groups or OA as a whole. Personal anonymity is maintained at the level of the media.

Since OA is not concerned with the medical aspects of obesity, it does not interfere with a physician's care.

OA offers five things to the compulsive overeater: acceptance, understanding, communication, relief, and power. If offers acceptance of you as you were, are, and will be. It understands the problems that you have and share with the other members of the group. Communication results from this mutual understanding. When you have found the first three, relief is found. Power is gained over your life, and a door to new behavior is opened.

In various publications, other guidelines are offered. You learn to weigh and measure your food. You write down a daily eating plan and report it to your sponsor. You avoid "binge" foods, eat slowly, sit down to eat,

119

weigh yourself once a month, and telephone other members for support when needed. Use of alcohol is discouraged. Other "tools" are provided to help you overcome the desire to take that "first bite" of a tempting food. Literature for every possibility is available. The tools and ideas are based on AA material.

The critical issue, as I see it, is that, while alcoholism and obesity are similar in some respects, they differ fundamentally. An AA "sponsor" needn't be an expert to tell others what to avoid, because there is only one prohibition—alcohol. Obesity calls for more professional treatment because the number of foods available to choose from is staggering. Also, you must eat to stay alive, while you can go without alcohol forever. So it becomes the problem of the compulsive overeater either to decide for himself which diet to follow, or to depend on someone else to decide for him.

On the basis of attending one meeting, I am certainly not going to judge Overeaters Anonymous. The psychological assistance it provides has undoubtedly helped many people. I would merely say that, in challenging obesity, the quality of outside help is a serious consideration. To trust the treatment of obesity to other sufferers exclusively can deny you important information. I endorse OA, but with the reservation that it treats only one part of the problem. I have discussed how a high-fat, high-sugar, low-fiber diet is dangerous to human beings. If you think this group could help you, try it, but be certain to combine OA's help with a generous amount of knowledge about nutrition.

13

Modern Vegetarianism

In the process of learning about nutrition as a way of controlling diabetes or weight, many of you will be exposed to vegetarianism. In this chapter, I would like to explain briefly what vegetarianism is, why it developed, and how to practice it safely and beneficially, should you choose to do so.

Vegetarianism, or abstaining from meat, fish, and fowl in the diet, with or without the use of dairy products and eggs, is not new. As early as Biblical times it was practiced (in some cases endured) because of food shortages or religious beliefs. In areas where animal foods were scarce, vegetarianism became a necessity for survival. Over the years, mixtures of foods that *were* available were developed to provide the best possible nutrition. Even back then, however, voluntary vegetarianism existed. Nowadays Trappist monks avoid meat because they consider it a luxury. Hindus will not eat meat because of their belief that the killing of an animal is the same as the killing of a man. Seventh Day Adventists avoid meat as an act of compassion and self-discipline. All these groups can be considered "traditional" vegetarians because their habits arise out of long-established religious practices.

There is a new and much larger group of vegetarians who for many reasons adopt a variety of meatless diets. The reasons can be either religious, ecological, economic, metaphysical, preferential, political, or health-oriented. These types are considered "new" because of

121

the many forms they take, and because the motivation for them is not based on either shortages or traditional religious beliefs.

There is no one diet which defines vegetarianism. The avoiding of red meat, fowl, and seafood is one. Pescovegetarians eat fish. Pollovegetarians eat fowl. Lactovegetarians add dairy products to their diets, while Lacto-ovo-vegetarians eat both dairy products and eggs. Vegans, one of the stricter types, use no animal products whatsoever, avoiding natural-bristle brushes, animal-based cosmetics and soaps, fur, wool, leather, silk, and pearls. Zen macrobiotics have a ten-step plan which progressively eliminates everything but brown rice.

Some small groups exist which could be called cults. The previously mentioned Zen macrobiotics follow the late George Ohsawa down the "path of longevity and peace of mind" through a belief in Zen and rigid dietary practices. Strictly following George has led some of his followers lemminglike over the cliff of health and into the chasm of malnutrition and early death. There is no single food that is complete enough to support life, and brown rice isn't even close.

Yoga followers avoid meat because they consider it near decomposition and a burden to the body. Also, since they believe in reincarnation, it's always possible to them that they and their domestic animals might be related. The members of the order of Sufi eat much as do Yoga followers.

The Ehrets Mucusless Diet Healing System is largely a fruitarian (fruit) diet. Its followers believe that meat causes mucus, which in turn breeds disease. All "new" vegetarians believe that they can purify their bodies and souls through vegetarianism.

Are You Circumscribed?

The above question indicates a way of categorizing vegetarians. Johanna T. Dwyer et al. classified vegetarians as circumscribed if they avoided three or fewer of the following five food groups: meat, poultry, fish and seafoods, eggs, and dairy foods. If they avoided four or five and also had extensive non-animal avoidances, they were called "far-reaching." She further divided the groups into "loners"—those not a member of any vegetarian group—and "joiners"—those belonging to a group which advocates vegetarianism. I like to call them CL's (circumscribed loners), CJ's (circumscribed joiners), and FJ's (far-reaching joiners). Far-reaching loners were rare and not prevalent enough to study.

When Dwyer et al. studied 100 "new" vegetarians, they found a wide spectrum of food use—from the avoidance of red meat only to the proscription of many foods. Dwyer's subjects were aged 17 to 35 and were 60 percent male. All weighed less than their highest adult weight. Thirty-six were "mild avoiders," having 1 to 2 avoidances out of the basic 5. Twenty-six had 3 avoidances, 15 had 4 or 5, and 23 were "vegans" who avoided all 5 categories of animal food. In men, extreme avoiders had more weight loss. Fifty-six persons lost weight on their vegetarian diet.

Some of the other characteristics of "new" vegetarians were as follows: 17 belonged to traditional religious groups, 43 belonged to philosophical or spiritual groups, and 58 based their diet on religious, spiritual, or philosophical convictions. Some of the other foods avoided by "new" vegetarians were legumes, cooked foods, cereals and grain, nonorganic food, processed food, canned food, frozen food, and additives. Twenty-eight used food supplements. Sixty-six thought that their diets were high in nutrition; only 13 felt that their diets were lacking in any nutrients. When asked their opinions about the medical profession, many wanted their physicians to be more sympathetic about vegetarianism and wanted more emphasis on prevention rather than on the curing of disease.

In another study done by Dwyer, her subjects' reasons for adopting vegetarianism and their group affiliations were explored. Out of 100 vegetarians, 35 gave health as their motivation. They felt that the diet improved their mental function and helped prevent health problems. Twenty-five subjects gave ethical reasons. They believed in nonviolence and the dignity of life. Fourteen gave metaphysical reasons. Vegetarianism helped them achieve spiritual balance and put them in the proper frame of mind for meditation. Eight gave ecology or a desire to prevent waste as their reason. Another 8 just didn't like meat. Three became vegetarian for economic reasons, 2 for religious, 2 for political, and 3 for curiosity or other reasons.

Dwyer found that CL's take more supplements. Joiners don't seek medical treatment as often. FJ's sometimes fast. Forty-three subjects thought some foods had medicinal qualities. Fifty-five felt that some foods were hazardous because of sugar, additives, or preservatives. Sixty-nine said that they planned to follow their diet indefinitely.

While loners tend to belong to traditional religions, joiners are more likely to belong to spiritual or philosophical groups and regard eating as a religious experience. Sixty-five percent of the subjects meditate or pray daily. Thirty-eight percent felt that their diet made them calmer, more spiritual, and clearer in thought.

Next, Dwyer turned her attention to preschool vegetarians. One hundred and sixty-three vegetarian parents volunteered 119 children under 5 years old. Breastfeeding status was determined by questioning.

Of the 119 subjects, 49 were macrobiotic, 24 were Yogic, 10 were Seventh Day Adventists, and 17 were not affiliated. The results of this study indicate that the children of vegetarians are lower in height, weight, and triceps skinfold than nonvegetarian children. After breast-feeding age, more vegetarian subjects' measurements were below average, and they were also leaner as a group. Basically, vegetarianism in children is associated with smallness, lightness, and leanness, and the stricter the diet, the more pronounced the characteristics.

Dwyer also points out that vegetarians in general often report loss of weight; greater regularity, frequency, and bulk in bowel functions; a positive state of mind; greater sensitivity to light, noise, and smell; a more pleasing body odor; less frequent sore throats and colds; decreased nervousness; fewer skin problems; fewer gas pains; greater hair growth; less hair brittleness and loss; and less dizziness.

Nutritional Implications

In order to better advise vegetarians, health professionals have studied vegetarian diets to determine their safety. Depending on the type and strictness of the diet, several problems can occur. The main problems have to do with calories, protein, vitamins, and minerals.

Vegetarian diets tend to be very high in bulk for their caloric content. Thus, it is sometimes hard for the vegetarian practitioner to eat enough food to fulfill his daily caloric requirements. When caloric needs aren't met, protein is used for energy (a very wasteful process), and protein needs increase.

Since animal foods are the only source of complete proteins, limiting your use of animal foods makes it harder to supply your body with protein. The human body needs nine different amino acids (proteins) for growth and repair. Most plant foods have only certain amino acids. We say that the quality of plant proteins is lower than that of animal proteins, but we mean that certain amino acids are missing from certain plants. To get high-quality (all amino acids) proteins, a vegetarian must mix several foods in his diet.

Dairy foods provide about 75 percent of the body's calcium needs and 39 percent of its need for riboflavin. If dairy products are not eaten, other sources of these nutrients must be found and used.

The high fiber content of a vegetarian diet may decrease absorption of certain minerals such as zinc or magnesium. Intake of these should be increased accordingly.

The only sources of vitamin D are egg yolk, butter, liver, some fish, and sunlight on the skin. Vitamin B_{12}

is another nutrient primarily of animal origin. Iron, found in meat and eggs, can also be deficient in an all-plant diet. Iodized salt should be used to provide iodine, which is found only in certain marine fish and shellfish.

Needed Nutrients

To be healthy, we must have certain nutrients every day. First of all, women need about 2,200 calories a day, while men need about 3,000. Every adult needs about 30 to 40 grams of protein to repair and replace lost cells. The vitamin requirements are shown in Table 13.1.

Table 13.1

Daily Nutrient Requirements for Adults

Vitamin A	1 mg.
Vitamin D	.01 mg.
Thiamine	1.5 mg.
Riboflavin	1.8 mg.
Niacin	20 mg.
Folicin	.4 mg.
B_{12}	.003 mg.
Vitamin C	45 mg.
Calcium	800 mg.
B_6	2 mg.
Pantothenic acid	5–10 mg.
Vitamin E	15 mg.
Vitamin K	.03 mg.
Iron	10 mg.
Phosphorus	800 mg.
Potassium	2500 mg.
Chlorine	2000 mg.
Sodium	2500 mg.
Magnesium	350 mg.
Fluorine	2 mg.
Zinc	15 mg.
Copper	2 mg.
Iodine	.14 mg.
Water	1.5 liters

Meeting these needs is fairly simple on a lacto-ovo-vegetarian diet. Milk and eggs in even moderate amounts combine with the incomplete grain and vegetable proteins to make a very satisfactory diet. Examples of dishes providing complete proteins would be beans and rice, macaroni and cheese, and cereal and milk. Wheat, for instance, is low in the amino acid lysine, but when combined with milk, it makes a complete protein. By eating three to four eggs per week and a cup of milk each day, one can correct any deficiencies in an otherwise varied and well-selected all-plant diet. One should also strive to decrease empty calories; eat legumes, nuts, and meat analogs; use low-fat milk products; and increase whole grains, fruits, and vegetables.

Strict Vegetarianism

Strict vegetarianism or veganism is the elimination of all animal products from the diet. The two main concerns of the vegan should be protein and vitamin B_{12} To supply adequate protein, foods must be eaten in proper combinations. Wheat can be combined with yeast, soybeans, nuts, or legumes. Peanuts supplement wheat, corn, oats, rice, and coconut. Soybeans supplement wheat, corn, and rye. Soy plus sesame resembles milk. Legumes and leafy vegetables supplement cereals. Vitamin B_{12} should be taken as a supplement, because there is no reliable plant source of this nutrient.

Since strict vegetarian diets are very high in bulk, it is often difficult to eat enough food to get a balanced diet. Some people find it hard just to get enough calories. If this is a problem for you, include some richer foods in your menu. If you eliminate milk, a good substitute is fortified soy milk with B_{12}, riboflavin, and calcium. Be sure to eat green leafy vegetables each day. You can use broccoli, brussels sprouts, collards, dandelion greens, kale, mustard greens, spinach, or turnip greens. A pure vegetarian diet that is sufficient in all nutrients except vitamin B_{12} can be selected.

The human body stores vitamin B_{12} in quantities a thousand times the recommended daily amount. Symptoms of deficiency, therefore, are rare, even after many years, but can occur when a vegan diet is followed by someone with malabsorption of B_{12} or a disorder causing an increased need for the vitamin.

Zen Macrobiotic Diet

This strict regimen is probably the most dangerous of all the vegetarian types. The follower is encouraged to drop first meat, fish, and fowl from the diet; later, dairy foods, eggs, vegetables, fruits; and finally everything but brown rice. This process is supposed to cleanse and purify the system of foreign substances. What it in fact does is limit the nutrition below life-supporting levels. In this diet protein, fat, vitamins, and minerals are so lacking that multiple deficiencies are sure to occur.

Symptoms Of Deficiency And Excess

While deficiencies and excesses happen only rarely, I'd like to mention them for your information and safety. Nevin S. Scrimshaw and Vernon R. Young have listed the symptoms of vitamin deficiency and excess, along with the recommended daily amounts, in the September 1976 issue of *Scientific American*. Deficiencies are much more dangerous and likely than excesses. For that reason supplements, chosen wisely, are cheap insurance for the vegetarian. The only nutrients for which excesses are a serious problem are Vitamin A, Vitamin D, and some of the trace minerals. If you feel that you get plenty of these, don't supplement. However, it is hardly likely that the amounts found in a multi-vitamin-mineral tablet would be harmful.*

* The following conditions can change your need for certain nutrients: acute or chronic infections, diseases, trauma, anxiety, fear, stress, kidney disease, intestinal parasites (tapeworm), or malaria. See your physician.

Raised levels of blood cholesterol carry a major risk for coronary heart disease. Several studies have looked at the effect of various vegetarian diets on cholesterol levels.

West et al. compared vegetarian and nonvegetarian Seventh Day Adventists, matched for place of residence, sex, age, marital status, height, weight, and occupation. All vegetarians over twenty-five had lower cholesterol levels than nonvegetarians.

In a population of 22 vegans and 22 omnivorous subjects, Sanders et al. found that weights, skinfold thicknesses, serum vitamin B_{12}, cholesterol, and triglycerides were all less in vegan subjects than in the controls. They concluded that a vegan-type diet may be the one of choice in the treatment of ischemic heart disease, angina pectoris, and certain hyperlipidemias.

Roland Phillips et al. made a six-year study of Seventh Day Adventists in California. They found that the coronary heart disease mortality rate for those who follow a lacto-ovo-vegetarian diet was only 28 percent of the rate for nonvegetarian Californians in the age group under 65, and 50 percent of the non-vegetarian rate for those over 65. While abstaining from alcohol and tobacco use is part of the reason for this reduced risk, at least half of the low risk is attributable to the vegetarian diet itself. Male Californian Adventists have their first heart attack an average of 10 years later than other male Californians. In general, a well-planned vegetarian diet could have side benefits of weight loss, lowered blood levels of cholesterol, lipids, lipoproteins, and triglycerides—all suspected of aggravating heart problems.

Recommendations

Vegetarianism per se is not a reason for concern. It is the extremity and type that are important. The more restrictive a diet is, the more dangerous it can be.

For adults following a strict vegetarian diet, several cautions are in order. Make sure that you get complete proteins by combining two or more incomplete plant proteins at the same meal. Supplement your diet with Vitamin B_{12}. Eat as much variety as you can—the more variety, the safer the plan. Use a soy meat-analog as a main course. Lacto-ovo-vegetarians have much less problem getting a balanced diet. Even a cup of milk a day and an egg every other day is sufficient to supplement a vegetarian diet. Variety in the grains, vegetables, fruits, and legumes is still necessary, however.

In children, the problems are a little greater. No child should be made to endure a Zen macrobiotic diet or any diet that allows only a few foods. Withholding milk and eggs from growing children is inadvisable. Growth can be stunted if certain nutrients are not available every day. I recommend that growing children get the following each day:

1 cup milk or fortified soy milk
1 cup legumes
20–30 grams textured vegetable protein
1.5 tablespoons nuts and seeds
4 tablespoons butter
.5 cup cooked fruit
1 cup raw fruit
.5 cup fruit juice
1 serving green leafy vegetables
1 serving vitamin-C-rich vegetables
1 slice whole-wheat bread
.5–.75 cup cooked cereal
1 egg
1 teaspoon fat
1.5 liters water

As in all diets, try to restrict sugars, refined foods, and alcohol. Please, parents, there is no other way your child can get these things if he doesn't eat them. For your child to eat the right foods, you have to provide them to the child in proper amounts and at proper times. Give some consideration to color, form, texture, and flavor, to avoid monotony. No other parental obligation is more important.

Justifications

There are some good reasons, both personal and global, for using fewer animal foods. On the personal side, weight can be lost, daily fat intake can be reduced, and the cost of food is sometimes less. There is no scientific way of distinguishing "organic" or "natural" foods from those at the grocery store. Therefore, if you pay more, you have to trust the farmer's or distributor's word that the foods are somehow different. By lowering your intake of fat and sugar, and increasing your dietary fiber, you may avoid diabetes, heart disease, obesity, and several diet-related cancers.

In the global context, leaning toward vegetarianism could fight hunger. On 1 acre of land, 13 pounds of protein can be produced if soybean, peas, or beans are the crop. If carrots, potatoes, califlower, brown rice, or cabbage are the crop, 4.2 pounds of protein are provided. But if poultry, beef, lamb, or pork is the crop, only 1.6 pounds of protein result. Plant protein is probably the food of the future—a time when tillable land will be at a premium.

14

Nutrition: Vitamins and Minerals

Nutrition is somewhat of a household word today; in fact, we hear it so often, we all perhaps feel that we humans have known about nutrition for a good long time, almost forever. Such is not the case—in fact, far from it! Scientific study of the requirements and elements of nutrition began less than a hundred years ago, and the word *vitamin* has been part of our vocabulary for less than seventy years.

Even today, how many understand its true meaning? We've all heard of vitamins, minerals, and nutrients—right? Of course we have, but do we comprehend their true significance to our health? While it is not important to most of us to understand how electricity works, it is significant to know that the light goes on when the switch is flipped. That is, we must know, at the very least, what happens to our bodies when various foods are eaten.

What Is Nutrition?

Nutrition is really two things—a science and a practice. The science of nutrition includes biochemistry, physiology, physics, and so forth—disciplines that deal with the biological system of man in relationship to what he eats. Nutrition as a practice belongs to the medical arts and includes sociological factors as related to food. I shall deal with nutrition both as a science and as a practice.

There will be those of you who will say, "What is he talking about? The nutrients required by our body have not changed over the years. Nutrition must be more than a hundred years old." That is true, very true. The required nutrients haven't changed, but something else has—our lifestyles and our associated diets are the culprits.

For example, look around you. What do you see? Automobiles everywhere! People walk less and less; they are not exercising. What is the result? Obesity— too many fat people driving those cars. Our lifestyles have changed, and not totally to the best interests of our health. Riding instead of walking reduced our need for calories, but the adjustment was not made. We learned to trade the car in when things started to go wrong, or technology upgraded the car, but few of us changed our diets as our body gave us signals to trade or change, and one such signal is being fat. Fat is the result of eating more calories than the body needs; the lifestyle was changed, the diet was not.

Does the presence of fat indicate that the body has or is receiving all the nutrients it needs? Not at all. Fat may indicate only a high-sugar, high-fat diet, for example. A third of our population are classified as obese, meaning that they are 20 percent over the standard of weight, according to actuarial charts. As I have stated in previous chapters, diabetes, high blood pressure, gall bladder disease are all related to obesity. A change in diet is manifestly necessary for survival.

Along with the changing technology in our world, we have seen other changes in addition to obesity. Where once rickets, scurvy, beri-beri, and pellagra were the scourges of man, there are now heart disease, cancer, arthritis, diabetes. The quality of the air we breathe and the water we drink has deteriorated; these factors themselves dictate a change in our diet.

All too often, where there has been a diet change it has been not positive but negative—junk foods, which cover our nation's tables. The root of many malignancies is to be found in nutrition. It is my firm belief that the main cause of death in our American civilization is what we voluntarily put in our mouths.

This daily "spoon and fork" debilitation may not produce visible results for many years, and perhaps that is why we are so oblivious to its insidious dangers. When it finally surfaces as heart disease, circulatory disorder, or cancer, years later, the daily misadventure with the spoon and fork is not suspect, let alone put to trial and convicted. Thus, nutritional killers are eminently more successful than the infectious diseases, which are soon recognizable and against which appropriate battles are then waged and won.

We must react to the alien toxic input into our bodies—and now. Tomorrow is always a day too late.

The Enemies

What must take place? The providing of proper nutrients to cells and tissue must occur on a continuing basis. We must strive not merely for "minimum" function, but for "maximum" function. Why be less than we can be? We have been, and will continue to be, what we eat!

While we frequently hear about a "balanced diet," few of us now in reality see or taste such a diet. Modern food-processing, shipping, storing, freezing, unfreezing, refreezing, cooking, refrigerating, reheating all take their toll on the foods on our plates. There is some food value still there, but much has vanished. Vitamins, sensitive to heat, light, air, and chemical processing, are the prime victims in our modern food. "Vitamin- and mineral-depleted food" is a more accurate description.

It is, of course, the vitamins and mineral content that completes the biochemical process of metabolism. The utilization of proteins, carbohydrates, and fats requires enzymes, and it is vitamins and minerals that are crucial to the functioning of specific enzymes. Thus, a deficiency of vitamins and minerals will affect proper metabolism.

Sugar has in it the sweetness of death. It is sweet by

no other name. It is devoid of vitamins, has a trace of minerals, and will not spoil—it has nothing of value left in it to spoil. But do not be deceived; if sugar cannot spoil, it can indeed be a "spoiler." Sugar can and will ruin your health. Yet it accounts for one-fourth of our daily calorie count. The long-term effect of sugar on our health is perhaps beyond measure. "Deadly sweet" would represent an accurate label.

Bleached flour and polished rice are other well-known vitamin-depleted victims of modern food-processing methods. An ounce of wheat germ contains 8 times the protein of 1 ounce of white flour. Does this ratio of 8 to 1 sound "balanced" to you? Of course not. Yet refined staples represent as much as one-half of our daily food intake.

Drying, canning, bleaching, boiling, deodorizing, and reconstituting all have an effect on our "balanced" diet—not in our favor. The milk we put on our cereal contains twice the protein and six times the calcium of the cereal itself. Some forms of roughage, such as cereals, may pay a very short visit to your body.

Potatoes picked in the fall lose one-fourth of their vitamins by spring, and almost all by summer. Apples and vegetables also suffer great losses of vitamins with each passing month. In most cases, it is months before these foods reach our tables. Therefore, vitamin loss is great and absolute. Calorie content is your only assurance, and that is not sufficient for proper body metabolism.

Long-term, subtle, but nevertheless inexorable suicide is a familiar daily picture; refined sugar and processed fruit juice for breakfast, several cups of coffee, a fast-food lunch—and, even worse, a martini to "wash it down"—more caffeine and a reheated meal for dinner. Sound familiar to any of you? For many, cigarettes are an added "dessert."

It is also to be noted here that even a dramatic turn-about in our dietary habits will not correct completely the long-term damage of bad nutrition, although it certainly would be a step on the road back to national good health. The truth is that even temporary nutritional deprivation has extended effects on our health, not just a "temporary effect." In essence, your future is the past, what you ate yesterday!

There is an ever-increasing case for nutritional wisdom and emphasis, which must of necessity incorporate vitamins into our diet planning. High-fiber foods, as I have already stressed, must also be specifically included in your daily meals. For if you are to plan and map your future, you must also plan your "daily bread."

General Rules

What can you do to maximize your future? Start today; every day counts. Avoid processed foods as much as possible. Stay away from sugar, white and brown, as if it were the plague. White flour and white rice have been stripped of much of their nutrient values and should not be used when you have a choice of whole-wheat bread and brown rice. Always eat the unrefined flours whenever possible.

Sun-ripened fruit and garden-fresh vegetables are preferred, but almost impossible for most of us to procure. For most of us, only the shipped and stored produce is available. Canned and frozen foods take their toll on vitamin content. To illustrate, cooking may reduce the vitamin C content of a fresh garden vegetable by 50 percent, whereas freezing that vegetable may cause a 60 percent loss, and canning an 80 percent loss.

Avoid reheating foods. Cook only enough for that particular meal, as vitamin content is reduced in the storing and reheating process. Stay away from the refined-cereal breakfast, as well as the cup of coffee and the cigarette.

Take care with your daily intake of salt. Use as little as possible, and whenever you can, do without it. Your health will be the better for it.

Food Supplements

Place yourself on a food supplement schedule of vitamins. As you do, bear in mind that there is no average vitamin requirement, because needs vary with each individual. Furthermore, the individual's daily need will fluctuate because each day's circumstances will change. Heat, light, alcohol, stress, aspirin, and chemicals destroy vitamins. The Recommended Dietary Allowance (RDA) published by the government does not take into consideration the individual's age, weight, sex, genetic structure, past medical history, or his/her environment. The RDA may meet only minimal needs at best.

While it is most difficult to tell each individual exactly what his/her vitamin intake should be, it is safe to say that your needs will vary and the RDA will probably not be sufficient to meet your daily needs. Please also bear in mind that not all the vitamins ingested are actually absorbed by the body. Internal losses occur, just as do external losses. For example, some vitamins may be locked in indigestible cells. You should also know that vitamins work as a team and that they are interdependent upon each other for correct metabolism. Protein, for example, requires A and B₃ for proper metabolism.

Further, the water-soluble vitamins, B-complex and C, cannot be stored in the body.

Pollutants play havoc with these vitamins, and adequate replacement is necessary to assure the body of correct metabolic processes. External pollutants, plus those self-imposed such as tranquilizers, barbiturates, sleeping pills, and alcohol demand that we have vitamin supplementation.

It behooves all to know that vitamins are not drugs and in fact are foods. Excess water-soluble vitamins are excreted and fat-soluble ones are stored for future use. Vitamins are our assurance of correct and optimal metabolic function, and optimal vitamin intake is heartily recommended. In this case, those levels recommended by Dr. Robert Benowicz in his book *Vitamins and You* are of high merit.

Abnormal situations, such as illness, surgery, pregnancy, and exceptional physical or emotional demands may call for increased supplementation, but only and always under the direction of a physician.

Nutrition in the Future

The decade of the '80s and beyond will see welcome changes in our dietary habits for several reasons. As the world population increases, we must seek cheaper and more abundant sources of protein. Meats polluted with drugs, antibiotics, and pesticides, and costing more and more, must give way to a less expensive and better source of protein, such as soybean products. Soya protein allows a fivefold increase in available protein over crop land used to feed cattle. Soya products such as soya flours and grits contain 50 percent protein. Soya protein concentrates contain 70 percent protein, and isolated soya proteins are over 90 percent protein! As of June 1980, the cost of vegetable protein was $0.70 per pound, compared to ground beef protein at $12.40 per pound. Yearly, 1 acre of land will yield a 77-day supply of beef for 1 person, wheat will yield an 877-day supply of wheat products, and soybeans on that same acre will provide food for 2,224 days for 1 person, an amazing difference!

Nutrition as related to aging in the 1980s and beyond merits special consideration. Today, life expectancy is 73 years, as compared to 47 years in 1900. More than 11 percent of our population is 65 or older, and by the year 2000 the figure will approach 25 percent. Of the people reading this book today, 80 percent can expect to see at least their seventieth birthday. A proper diet greatly enhances that likelihood.

It is a fact that a number of the health problems associated with advancing years have their roots in earlier years of poor nutrition. As I have indicated, and proved over and over, poor dietary habits cause not only obes-

138

ity and diabetes but many other ailments as well. I must again stress that temporary nutritional deprivation has long-term effects on our bodies. Every day of good nutrition counts, as well as every day of poor nutrition. The evidence is strong that past vitamin depletion can raise present metabolic needs on a continuing basis.

In Your Later Years

As we continue to age, our nutritional requirements change. The aging process itself differs in every individual as to rate and degree, but it is constant and must be accounted for.

For example, the metabolic rate slows about 16 percent during the 30-to-70 age span. Advancing years reduce calorie requirements by 33 percent; our bodies tell us that, if we listen to the messages, which most of us do not. However, as the calorie requirements reduce with age, be aware that the vitamin and good nutrition needs do not!

Vitamin need increases with advancing age. You must make certain that as the protein molecules decrease in your body there are sufficient supplies of vitamin co-enzymes. Also, as the amount of physical activity decreases and food intake correspondingly decreases, the need for vitamin supplementation increases.

Other factors to be dealt with in advancing age are chewing and swallowing difficulties, poor digestion, and interference by various drugs. All accentuate the necessity for vitamin intake to meet the nutritional need, which is undiminished.

Preparation for old age really should begin with yesteryear—in childhood. Children should eat wholesome food, not snacks, processed substitutes, and the various junk foods that inundate the market. It is usually later in life that the consequences of what goes into the body system surface. Such a vision is not a "picture of health." Youth can no longer mask the consequences of a faulty diet. The debt must be paid!

As the preparation for a long and healthy life surely begins with youth, good nutrition must begin with good digestion, for indeed digestion is at the river's beginning of nutritional flow.

Digestion is the process by which food is prepared for absorption in the body. The nutrients are then later absorbed through the small intestine.

As foods consist of long chains of molecules, they must be chopped up, rearranged, and changed in molecular composition so that the body may properly use food nutrients. Such changing and rearranging is brought about by enzymes, which are proteins formed in the body from amino acids. Each enzyme acts on a certain type of substance to bring about the changes required by our body. Proteins, vitamins, and minerals are needed for the making of digestive enzymes.

Enzymes that act on protein will not act on fat or carbohydrates, and there is an enzyme that will split protein molecules; enzymes are that specific. Enzymes are found in both plant and animal tissue cells and are usually named for their functions. For example, "lipases" are fat-splitting enzymes, named from the word "lipids" for fats. Vitamins are known to assume the task of co-enzymes and act as catalysts, as well as taking part in enzymatic reactions.

Enzymes convert protein to amino acids, fat to fatty acids, and carbohydrates to simple sugars. These compounds are then absorbed as they pass through the lining of the intestine into the blood. Such absorption is not the same for all of us, and can be assisted or inhibited by various nutrients, as well as by mental states. Thus, poor nutrition will make its negative presence known in the digestive process, and if inadequate nutrients are supplied to the body, natural functioning will be inhibited. Specific nutrients, then, are essential and vital to our good health, and vitamins play an important role in our daily well-being.

Balance—the Proteins

The amino acids, converted from protein by enzymes, number twenty, of which eleven are nonessential. The nine essential amino acids are isoleucine, leucine, lysine, methionine, phenylalanine, threonine, tryptophan, valine, and histidine. When these acids are in their proper proportion, the body can build tissue protein, and so it is that "balanced" protein foods are called "complete protein foods." Large quantities of protein are therefore not as important as "complete" or "balanced" proteins.

The more we know of life, the more we learn of nature's need for balance. It is proper balance in all things for which we should strive. When that is achieved, there is a harmony of functions, actions, and interactions.

Balance—the Carbohydrates

Carbohydrates are part of the balancing team. They too are chains that must be broken down by enzymes for body use. Carbohydrate chains are usually simple sugars, water-soluble, and are stored in different ways. Monosaccharides, or simple sugars, are found in fruit and vegetable plants and include glucose, fructose, and galactose. Simple sugars are stored as starch, which is broken down to glucose units before use by the body. As starch is broken down into glucose, dextrin and maltose sugars are formed by the process. Combinations of two sugars are called disaccharides; sucrose is such a combination.

Glycogen is simple sugar stored in the liver, which also must be broken down to glucose before it can be used by the body as quick energy.

Carbohydrates make us fat when we consume more than we need. As we eat more carbohydrates than the body requires in the form of glucose, and more than can be stored in the form of glycogen, the excess is converted to fat and stored in adipose (fat) tissue.

Balance—the Fats

Everybody needs fat; it is the balance or amount of fat in our body that is critical. Fat, combined with protein, lines the intestines, sheathes new cells, makes brain tissue, protects the body from undue loss of heat, protects organs from injury, and acts as a storage vehicle for energy. Excessive amounts of fats, such as cholesterol floating in the bloodstream, can block or impede circulation and cause a stroke or heart attack.

Excellent sources of carbohydrates are dried fruits, grains, legumes, and potatoes. Whatever the source, they are chains of simple sugars that are broken down into glucose for quick sources of energy.

Again, vitamins are essential for the carbohydrate metabolic process, with the B-complex vitamins front and center. The B vitamins also split molecules to make other compounds, as well as create molecular movements.

Balance—the Minerals

We cannot speak of balance in the world of nutrition without mentioning the role of minerals in the total process. Minerals act as the catalysts for the vitamins to trigger the enzymes into action. They are a vital food supplement, but they must be consumed with caution, as they can be toxic in excessive amounts. It is best not to exceed RDA specifications.

Without minerals, such nutrients as vitamins, protein, carbohydrates, and fat would be wasted. The macroinorganic minerals present in fairly large amounts in our bodies are calcium, phosphorus, magnesium, sodium, and potassium. The trace minerals, those found in smaller amounts, are chromium, copper, iodine, manganese, molybdenum, selenium, and zinc.

Calcium triggers enzyme reactions, is needed for nerve transmission, and, along with sodium, potassium, and magnesium, maintains the heart muscles and body muscle tone. Without it, blood would not clot, so the blood level of calcium is very important.

Magnesium, another enzyme activator, assists in the formation of adenosine triphosphate, often referred to as the "dynamite energy" of the body. It is needed to regulate body temperature, nerve impulses, and muscle contractions.

Potassium maintains the balance of all fluids and the body's acid-alkaline balance. It is also crucial in regulating heartbeat. Fruit lovers will be glad to hear that bananas, cantaloupes, and dried dates are excellent sources of potassium.

Phosphorus, with calcium, strengthens bone tissue and assists in cell division, as well as in transporting fats and fatty acids.

Sodium assists in balancing all fluids and the acid-alkaline levels. This is usually the one mineral we consume too much of, as salt is 40 percent sodium.

Zinc assists in the synthesis of new blood cells and in the digestive process. It is essential for the normal development of sex glands. Selenium appears to protect cell membranes, and manganese is vital to the synthesis of complex carbohydrates in cells, in utilization of glucose, and in muscle contraction.

Iron is well known for its ability to carry oxygen through the body. It is also important for tissue and cellular respiration. Although iron is the most common and cheapest of all nutrients, it is the most deficient nutrient in the American diet. This is because of the small amount of dietary iron actually absorbed by the body. For example, such rich sources of iron as raisins and spinach contain phytate and oxalate acids, which bind so rigidly with iron that bioavailability is very low.

Iodine is used by the healthy thyroid gland to produce thyroxine, which mostly determines the rate at which nutrients are supplied to our body. It is also required for carrying oxygen into the cells.

Minerals, then, are no small matter in the world of

nutrition. When selecting supplements, read the labels carefully to determine which minerals are included and in what amounts. They are vitally important to you.

I must repeat that good nutrition *must* be considered an integral part of your daily life, so that the number of your days, as well as the quality, can be maximized. It behooves you to bear in mind, that an overfed body may not be a well-nourished body. If you wish to lead an active, vigorous life into your seventies and eighties, follow a lifelong plan of good nutrition. The "golden harvest" years can only be golden for those who plant and tend the seed with proper care and diligence. A bountiful harvest almost never happens by accident, but by careful design.

15

Sample Menus for Renewed Health for Obese and Diabetic People

Please read this instruction: Before using these menus, consult your physician. He will guide and advise you.

1100 Calories
Low-fat, low-meat, high-fiber menu

BREAKFAST
¾ c. oatmeal with
2 Tbsp. apple fiber
1 high-fiber muffin
½ c. strawberries
4 oz. skim milk

LUNCH
Tofu egg salad—¼ lb. tofu
    4 tsp. imitation mayonnaise
    ¼ stalk celery, diced
    2 Tbsp. minced onion
    2 Tbsp. minced green pepper
Cabbage salad—1 c. shredded cabbage
    4 tsp. chopped onion
    4 tsp. chopped green pepper
    2 tsp. vinegar
    1 tsp. vegetable oil
    sugar substitute to taste
1 medium pear

DINNER
Stir-fried chicken—2 oz. chicken without skin
    ⅓ c. chopped bok choy
    2/3 c. peas
½ c. brown rice
½ c. steamed spinach
1 c. melon balls
4 oz. skim milk

145

SNACK   1 medium orange

Calories	1120
Protein	55.3 g.—19.8%
Carbohydrate	161.4 g.—57.6%
Fat	29.5 g.—23.7%
Fiber	14.5 g.
Cholesterol	68 mg.
Sodium	748 mg.

1200 Calories
Low-fat, low-meat, high-fiber menu

BREAKFAST   ¾ c. oatmeal with
2 Tbsp. apple fiber
1 high-fiber muffin
½ c. strawberries
8 oz. skim milk

LUNCH   Tofu egg salad—¼ lb. tofu
4 tsp. imitation mayonnaise
¼ stalk celery, diced
2 Tbsp. minced onion
2 Tbsp. minced green pepper
Cabbage salad—1 c. shredded cabbage
4 tsp. chopped onion
4 tsp. chopped green pepper
2 tsp. vinegar
1 tsp. vegetable oil
sugar substitute to taste
1 medium pear

DINNER   Stir-fried chicken—2 oz. chicken without
skin
1/3 c. chopped bok choy
2/3 c. peas
½ c. brown rice
½ c. steamed spinach
1 c. melon balls
8 oz. skim milk

SNACK   1 medium orange

Calories	1209
Protein	63.3 g.—20.9%
Carbohydrate	173.3 g.—57.3%

146

Fat	29.9 g.—22.2%
Fiber	14.5 g.
Cholesterol	73 mg.
Sodium	876 mg.

1500 Calories
Low-fat, low-meat, high-fiber menu

BREAKFAST
¾ c. oatmeal with
2 Tbsp. apple fiber
1 high-fiber muffin
½ c. strawberries
8 oz. skim milk

LUNCH
1 whole-wheat bagel
Tofu egg salad—¼ lb. tofu
    4 tsp mayonnaise
    ¼ stalk celery, diced
    2 Tbsp. minced onion
    2 Tbsp. minced green pepper
Cabbage salad—1 c. shredded cabbage
    4 tsp. chopped onion
    4 tsp. chopped green pepper
    2 tsp. sugar substitute to taste
    2 tsp. vinegar
    1 tsp. vegetable oil
1 medium pear

DINNER
Stir-fried chicken—2 oz. chicken without skin
    1/3 c. chopped bok choy
    2/3 c. peas
½ c. brown rice
½ c. steamed spinach
1 c. melon balls
8 oz. skim milk

SNACK
1 medium orange

Calories	1477
Protein	69.2g.—18.7%
Carbohydrate	213.8g.—57.9%
Fat	40.8g.—24.9%
Fiber	15 g.
Cholesterol	79 mg.
Sodium	1373 mg

2000 Calories
Low-fat, low-meat, high-fiber menu

BREAKFAST
½ c. strawberries
¾ c. oatmeal
1 slice whole-wheat French toast with
½ c. unsweetened applesauce and
2 Tbsp. apple fiber
8 oz. skim milk

LUNCH
1 whole-wheat bagel
Tofu egg salad—¼ lb. tofu
   4 tsp. mayonnaise
   ¼ stalk celery, diced
   2 Tbsp. minced onion
   2 Tbsp. minced green pepper
Cabbage salad—1 c. shredded cabbage
   4 tsp. chopped onion
   4 tsp. chopped green pepper
   2 tsp. sugar substitute to taste
   2 tsp. vinegar
   1 tsp. vegetable oil
1 medium pear

maple syrup ?→ (handwritten note)

DINNER
Stir-fried chicken—2 oz. chicken without
   skin
   1/3 c. chopped bok choy
   2/3 c. peas
¾ c. brown rice
½ c. steamed spinach
1 c. melon balls
2 slices whole-wheat bread
8 oz. skim milk

SNACK
1 high-fiber muffin
1 medium orange
½ c. yogurt, skim-style, with
½ c. blueberries and
3 Tbsp. apple fiber

Calories	1956
Protein	88.3 g.—18%
Carbohydrate	303 g.—62.0%
Fat	47.4 g. 218%
Fiber	26.2 g.
Cholesterol	192 mg.
Sodium	2104 mg.

2500 Calories
Low-fat, low-meat, high-fiber menu

BREAKFAST
2/3 c. Corn Bran® cereal
½ c. strawberries
½ c. bananas
1 slice French toast (use whole-wheat bread) with
½ c. unsweetened applesauce
1 high-fiber muffin
8 oz. skim milk

LUNCH
Spinach salad—3½ oz. raw spinach
   1 hard-cooked egg
   5 small raw mushrooms
   2 Tbsp. chopped onion
   2 Tbsp. herb and buttermilk dressing
1 c. bean soup
5 Ry-Krisp ® crackers
½ c. bananas with
1 c. skim yogurt and
4 Tbsp. apple fiber
2 slices whole-wheat bread

DINNER
Crustless cauliflower and carrot quiche—
   1/6th of pie
½ c. peas and mushrooms
½ c. wheat salad
8 oz. skim milk
1/9th of apple crisp (approx. ½ c.)
Fruit salad—½ med. apple, sliced with skin
   ¼ c. diced celery
   ¼ c. Thompson grapes

SNACK
1 whole pink grapefruit
1 c. popcorn (no fat or salt)
1 medium orange
2 large carrots

Calories	2453
Protein	97.7 g.—15.9%
Carbohydrate	371.7g.—60.6%
Fat	63.2g.—23.3%
Fiber	35 g.
Cholesterol	499 mg.
Sodium	3774 mg.

High-Fiber Raisin Muffins
(Makes 12 muffins)

1 cup all-purpose flour
1½ cups whole-wheat flour
1/3 cup corn oil
1/3 cup honey
2 teaspoons baking powder
1 egg
1 cup milk
2 cups raisins
¾ cup oatmeal
1 cup hot water
1 cup wheat bran

Mix all ingredients together into dough. Add wheat bran last. Put into muffin tins and cook at 350° for 20 to 30 minutes, or until brown.

Each muffin contains:

Carbohydrate	37.2 grams
Fat	8.4 grams
Protein	6.9 grams
Crude fiber	1.5 grams
Calories	249

Soybean-Corn-Tomato Casserole
(12 servings)

2½ cups cooked soybeans
1½ cups canned corn, drained
2 tablespoons flour
1 teaspoon sugar
1 teaspoon garlic salt
¼ teaspoon Basil leaves
¼ teaspoon pepper
1 cup breadcrumbs
½ cup shredded Cheddar cheese
2 tablespoons butter

Mix soybeans and corn together. Mix flour, sugar, garlic salt, basil, pepper, and breadcrumbs together. Sprinkle on top of corn and soybean mixture. Top with shredded cheese and dot with butter. Cook for 1-1½ hours at 350°.

Wheat Salad
(makes 6 servings)

½ cup finely crushed bulgar
1 cup water
1 cup finely chopped fresh parsley
½ cup onion
1 medium fresh tomato chopped
3 tablespoons fresh lemon juice
3 tablespoons salad oil
½ teaspoon salt
¼ teaspoon black pepper
lettuce

Soak bulgar in water for ½ hour. Drain well. Add vegetables. Mix lemon juice, oil, salt, and pepper. Add to salad. Toss lightly to coat ingredients. Refrigerate 24 hours. Serve on lettuce leaves.

16

Most Commonly Asked Questions and Answers on Obesity, Diet, and Diabetes

Q. What is your "discovery"?

A. I have determined that 91.4 percent of adult-onset diabetes is due to diet, 8 percent is due to heredity, and 0.6 percent is due to environment. A diet high in fat, low in fiber, and high in sugar promotes the formation of excessive amounts of the female hormone—estrogen—which blocks the estrogen receptors in the hypothalamus, pituitary, and liver, and causes diabetes.

Q. Oh, good! Since I don't take estrogen, I won't get diabetes—right?

A. Wrong! Even people who don't take extra estrogen can be making their own.

Q. How?

A. Fat tissue and bacteria in your digestive tract can both make it.

Q. Why do some people make too much estrogen?

A. A diet high in fat and simple sugars and low in fiber and complex carbohydrates stimulates bacteria to make estrogen. Most Americans eat this type of diet.

Q. But I have always thought that diabetes was hereditary.

A. So did everyone, until now. I can show that 90 percent of adult-onset diabetes is due to diet.

Q. How is that?

A. A normal person's hypothalamus, pituitary, and liver have receptors for the hormone estradiol, which helps control insulin and metabolism. The excess hormone—estrone—that I was talking about sticks to these receptors and confuses the feedback system. The tissues become insensitive to insulin, and the level of sugar in the blood rises—causing diabetes.

Q. Well, I don't know. Has this theory been tested?

A. Yes, indirectly. For about a decade researchers in several countries, including one in Kentucky, have been treating diabetics with a high-fiber, high-carbohydrate, low-fat diet, with fantastic results. Many diabetics can reduce the amount of their medications or their insulin, and some can eliminate them altogether.

Q. What are the risks?

A. None—with one condition. Don't try to change your medication without your doctor's supervision. The diet is safe for all people—diabetic or not.

Q. My doctor has never heard of this treatment. What should I tell him?

A. This is common. Tell your doctor that you want to try a high-fiber, high-carbohydrate, low-fat diet. Tell him you would like to see him frequently during this period, in case you need to change your insulin dosage. Tell him that it is a new approach, and offer to show him this book.

Q. What is wrong with the American diet?

A. We eat too much fat and sugar. Our diet is low in fiber. Our foods are too processed.

Q. There are lots of diets. What's so great about yours?

A. Most popular diets are aimed at temporary weight loss, whereas mine is aimed at permanent control of obesity and near normalization of blood sugar and diabetic symptoms.

Q. How does your diet accomplish all these things?

A. By lowering calories from fat intake from 42 percent to between 20 and 25 percent. By lowering sugar intake from 15 percent to 5 percent. By increasing carbohydrate intake from 48 percent to 60 percent.

Q. We get 42 percent of our calories as fat?

A. That's right, in steak, pork, french fries . . .

Q. Do you eat pork at all?

A. Yes, in limited quantities. Chicken and fish are better.

Q. What do you think of vegetarian diets?

A. If balanced, they are fine.

Q. How about eggs?

A. Even with the fat and cholesterol, an egg contains 90 calories of pretty good food. Limit eggs to about 6 per week. Don't cook them in fat.

Q. What are complex carbohydrates?

A. Basically, grains, fruits, and vegetables.

Q. O.K., what are the simple ones, then?

A. Sugars—sucrose, dextrose, fructose, and syrups.

Q. Can I use honey, molasses, and brown sugar?

A. Not if you aren't supposed to have sugar, because they are all sugar.

Q. How many calories should I eat?

A. Enough to keep your body weight within 15 percent of your ideal body weight according to the Metropolitan Life Insurance tables. Never consume less than 600 calories per day unless you are on a medically supervised diet.

Q. Can I have coffee and tea?

A. They stimulate the production of urine and can cause irregular glucose levels. Try to limit them by substituting herb tea or juices.

Q. What about saccharine?

A. It is better for obese persons and diabetics than sugar. Moderation, please.

Q. How much fiber do I need?

A. About twenty grams of crude fiber per day.

Q. How many slices of wheat bread would that be?

A. About two hundred. You're going to have to make an effort here. Buy some wheat bran, soy bran, or apple bran, and add it to everything you can. Eat any fruit and vegetable skins that are palatable. Look for "whole grains" on labels, and you'll be on the right track.

Q. What about low-calorie sugar?

A. No such thing.

Q. Diet ice cream?

A. Poison.

Q. Does cooking destroy fiber?

A. Not usually. Some things—carrots for example—are better eaten raw.

Q. The rest of my family doesn't have diabetes. Can they eat this diet, too?

A. You mean they don't have diabetes *now*. By all means start feeding them right immediately. They'll last longer.

Q. If you are from India, how did you become diabetic on that very un-Western diet?

A. Good question! I got diabetes *after* I came to the United States and started eating steaks, bacon, and meatballs.

Q. But I thought that your father had diabetes in India.

A. Boy, you are sharp! You see, in India we were wealthy. Over there, wealthy people can afford all the "delicacies" Americans eat. So he got diabetes that way. At that time, I didn't know the cause.

Q. Should I take vitamins?

A. By all means. Especially if you are trying to lose weight. The less you eat, the harder it is to get all the nutrients you need.

Q. My sister's stepdaughter, age seven, has diabetes. Can she get off insulin with this diet?

A. No. You see, she is very likely to have juvenile-onset diabetes (type 1). About 5 percent of diabetics are in this category. Their pancreases do not make insulin, and therefore these persons can't follow my approach. Fortunately, the other 95 percent of diabetics have the adult-onset type (type 2). Their pancreases make an excess of insulin. If they get rid of the surplus estrogens in their systems, their insulin can go back to work.

Q. At what ages do you get the juvenile type?

A. Two to fourteen. Rarely as late as fifteen to twenty-four.

Q. Some juvenile diabetics are not fat. How do they get diabetes?

155

A. You've got me there. Some think that a crisis, such as an infection, shuts the pancreas down for good. The diet does help juvenile diabetics avoid the complications of diabetes. They will usually always need insulin, though.

Q. So how many diabetics are there, anyway?

A. About fifteen million total, with less than a million juveniles.*

Q. What is a "normal" blood-sugar count?

A. Between 70 and 110. Diabetics go from 200 to 3,000!

Q. Do your bowel habits give any indication of your health?

A. Yes. Populations with no risk for diabetes have large, soft stools, frequent clearing, and fast transit times. If you have small, hard stools, infrequent movements, and slow transit times (36 to 48 hours), you aren't eating enough fiber. You intestinal bacteria have more time to make the estrogens out of bile acids.

Q. Can thin adults still get diabetes?

A. Yes. A diet high in fat is a feast for the intestinal bacteria, even if the person doesn't gain weight.

Q. Do I understand correctly that the diet not only prevents diabetes but can cure it in certain circumstances?

A. Yes and no. Eating this way can prevent one from getting adult-onset diabetes. After that we get into trouble with definitions. Only extremely rarely is a diabetic ever "cured" of his disease. He can be symptom-free if he sticks to the diet, but he can never go back to his old eating habits. Think of the "cured" diabetic as similar to a reformed alcoholic. He's fine as long as he doesn't touch the "forbidden fruit."

Q. Isn't my "exchange" diet good enough?

A. No. It is probaby too high in fat. Check it over and see. I know that it is difficult, but try to determine if fat calories represent about 25 percent of the calories and carbohydrates about 60 to 70 percent. Also check

* Estimates for U.S.A., summer 1981.

156

to see if it includes 20 grams of crude fiber per day. Consult a dietitian if necessary. That's cheaper than seeing a doctor or having a terminal case of diabetes.

Q. Is diabetes aggravated by stress?

A. It can be. Often stress pushes the chemical diabetic over the borderline into clinical or measurable diabetes. If you eat properly, you won't be so close to the line and will be able to handle stress with no problems.

Q. Should diabetics exercise?

A. Yes. Exercise helps the tone of their muscles. To be effective, however, it must be combined with proper nutrition.

Q. I've heard that nutrition is responsible for many of our present leading causes of death. Can that be true?

A. Yes. In addition to diabetes, cancer of the bowel, breast, uterus, and prostate are all related to diet. Also, hypertension and other cardiovascular ailments can be prevented or postponed by good eating habits.

Q. Is hypoglycemia the same as diabetes?

A. Curiously, even though functional hypoglycemia is the *opposite* of diabetes, it is an early stage of diabetes. It means low blood sugar and is usually defined as being below 40–50, with 70–110 as normal.

Q. How do you get functional hypoglycemia?

A. Some people's pancreases are more sensitive to stimulation than others. After years of the typical American breakfast of coffee, doughnuts, and cigarettes (caffeine, sugar, nicotine—I see you smiling), the pancreas starts making more insulin than is needed. Blood-sugar level drops, and you feel lousy. You eat more of the same thing—a vicious cycle. It's not that simple, but you get the idea.

Q. So everything I like is bad for me. Where do you get the will power?

A. Look, it took a long time to get into this fix; take a little time and effort getting out of it. Every time you are tempted, ask yourself, "Is this going to be good for me or not?" Don't change drastically, but slowly. Get family and friends behind you.

157

Q. If estrogens are bad for you, why do doctors prescribe them?

A. They are currently rethinking this problem. Estrogens are useful for certain women for whom the threat of menopause-related ailments is greater than the threat of cancer or diabetes. For the majority, they are best avoided. In England, estrogens are prohibited.

Q. Aren't birth control pills made of estrogen?

A. Yes. And if you read the warnings on the package, you will notice that many of the problems have to do with metabolism, weight gain, and other things related to diabetes. Use something else.

Q. The doctors gave me estrogen before I had breast cancer.

A. I see. Well, we have a living example here.

Q. I am not worried about estrogens because I never took any.

A. Don't forget that a woman's body makes estrogens in many ways—the placenta, the ovaries, the adrenals, and possibly the intestines and fat tissue. You can prevent the last two by proper diet and weight loss.

Q. Wow! My diabetes started at the same time as my hysterectomy. I was given hormones because of that. If I stop the hormones, will my diabetes go away?

A. Slow down. When was your hysterectomy? If your diabetes started recently, and you have no permanent damage, the diet will fix you up. If your diabetes started ten to twenty years ago, and you have vascular damage, your condition can be improved but not restored.

Q. Could the added estrogen in obese women prevent them from conceiving?

A. It is possible that too much estrone compared with estradiol could increase the odds against conception. You have to have a balance.

Q. My husband and I are both overweight. Lately we've had trouble . . . he works a lot . . . he's always . . . maybe I've lost . . . he's a good provider . . . it used to be O.K., . . . what I'm trying to say is . . .

A. Your sex life is down the tube? Remember that estrogen is a *female* hormone. When a man has an excess, it affects his libido or sex drive. In a way, you could call my diet a "sex diet," because it could restore a normal sex drive to both sexes.

Q. Are you saying that my sex drive is abnormal?

A. Since estrogen is a female hormone, it tends to increase yours. I don't mean to say that you are a fiend. Just that at this time you need extra affection, and your husband possibly can't give it.

Q. HELP!!!

A. Eat less fat, less sugar, more fiber, and lose weight.

Gentlemen's Questions and Answers

Q. How dare you say that I have female hormones? Why, you dirty . . .

A. Just a minute. *All* men have some estrogens. It's just that obesity and high-fat diets cause an unusually high proportion of estrogens.

Q. Could this affect my . . . er . . .

A. Yes. For ten years I had this problem. My wife threatened divorce. Luckily, I made my discovery in time and reversed my hormonal imbalance through diet.

Q. But if an excess of estrogens decreases my sex drive, what does it do to the ladies?

A. It increases theirs.

Q. Great! Why change it, though?

A. Do you want your wife running around all day with an abnormally high sex drive? Seriously, couples will get along much better if both partners' sex drive is normal. My wife's diabetes has been normalized, and she retains a normal interest in sex.

Q. I recently lost weight but did not see the increase in sex drive.

159

A. Your reducing diet was low in calories but was not a high-fiber, low-fat diet. Even though you lost weight, your intestinal bacteria are still making estrogens.

Q. Is impotence common?

A. There are over 6,000 sexual dysfunction clinics in the United States. You tell me.

Q. But is impotence always caused by diet and diabetes?

A. No. But 50 to 70 percent of diabetic men are impotent. About 12 percent of impotent men are diabetic.

Q. O.K., I have to change my eating habits. Where do I get the will power?

A. Whenever I'm faced with a big, tempting meal, I ask myself, "Sam, do you want sex or diabetes?" The answer is usually quite easy.

Questions and Answers on Diet and Your Weight

In 1976, a Gallup Poll showed that 88 percent of American adults wanted to know more about nutrition. A Harris Poll found that only 14 percent of them thought that Americans ate a proper diet. Recent evidence of a decreasing incidence in deaths due to cardiovascular disease is encouraging news that our interest in nutrition is more than superficial. How much credit is due to improvements in diet, however, and how much is due to exercise programs or screening and treatment of hypertension is not known. But we do know that Americans are now more interested in their health and diet than in the past. Here are some questions commonly asked about nutrition, diet, and weight management.

Q. What is wrong with the American diet?

A. Generally, the problem lies with the excesses. Americans need to moderate their eating and drinking habits. Large amounts of any food or drink are bad for us. Small amounts are good. That's the safest and most practical solution anyone has found. Addiction to fast-fried foods, chocolates, and alcohol leads to consumption of excessive calories. Excessive calories lead to overweight, emotional disorders, and a host of other health problems. Since the leading causes of death in America are cardiovascular disorders, our greatest concern is the increased risk of heart attacks and strokes. But, regardless of how it affects our health, excess fat does not look good on us. It is fashionable in America to be slender. But attempts to become slender often lead to more problems than they solve. Not least are the expenses involved in "quick" weight-loss plans and concoctions.

Q. How can we solve the problem?

A. Most important is that we avoid abruptly altering our eating habits by adopting nutritionally deficient or unbalanced diets. Crash programs are often successful in the short term. But the rebound phenomena, whereby the dieter gains back the weight he lost and overshoots that mark, ending up fatter than before he started dieting, is not uncommon. Unsupervised exercise programs, too, have their faults, as witnessed by the number of new clinics for treatment of "sports injuries." Moderate changes are usually safe, but drastic changes in our lifestyles require expert supervision. So the safest answer is to exercise moderately, cut out all "junk foods" and alcoholic beverages, and see your doctor before making any extreme changes in your style of living.

Q. Why do I put on weight so easily, while others eat whatever they want and never gain a pound?

A. For most cases, there is a very simple explanation: More calories are consumed than the body is capable of utilizing. The excess calories are stored as fat. Individuals vary a great deal in the rate at which they utilize energy, or their metabolic rate. It is possible for two people who appear almost identical in other respects to eat identical diets. Yet one gets fat and the other stays slim. A person becomes overweight because his calorie intake exceeds his or her metabolic rate. A 2,000-calorie-per-day intake matched with a 1,500-calorie-per-day metabolic rate will result in an excess of 500 calories per day. This may not seem like much, but

3,500 calories produce about 1 pound of fat. In one week, one can gain 1 pound. Over a period of one year, this means an excess of 52 pounds.

Age is important. Our metabolic rate falls as much as 1 percent a year after age 35. If our need at that age is 2,500 calories, it will be 2,250 at age 45. If we continue to eat the same amount of food as we did 10 years earlier, we will gain ½ pound per week, or 26 pounds a year. If we continue the same regimen at age 55, we will gain one pound a week, or 52 pounds per year.

Q. How do I know that my excess weight is not due to something wrong with my glands?

A. One obese (excessively overweight) person in twenty (5 percent) has a thyroid problem. Your doctor can determine that possibility by a test that measures the level of thyroxine in your blood. In past years, it was necessary to measure your metabolic rate by testing your oxygen consumption. Then the "PBI" (protein-bound iodine) test was developed. Both oxygen consumption and the PBI test were rather crude, inaccurate measurements. We now use a radioimmuno-assay for thyroxine, a much more accurate test than either of the older procedures.

Q. What is my desirable weight?

A. Your desirable weight depends upon several variables—your body type, musculature, etc. Unless you have been fat all your life, your most desirable weight may be what you weighed at age twenty-five. If you are athletic, you can be overweight by the charts and still have no excess fat. Skinfold thickness is the best approximate measure of your body composition. As a rough estimate, we use data collected by the insurance companies to judge desirable weights for sex, height, body build, and age. Table 16.1 will help you establish a weight goal. Recent studies, however, have suggested that these data are too rigid. Unless you are 10 percent overweight by these charts, you do not necessarily have a weight problem. If you do not like the looks of yourself in the mirror and your wardrobe no longer fits, maybe all you need is an exercise program to tone your muscles and decrease the amount of fat in your body.

Q. What kind of exercise is best for weight management?

A. If you are excessively overweight, only moderate exercise (walking, bicycling, or swimming) is recommended. If you are less than twenty pounds overweight, exercise alone may be the answer, as long as you don't reward yourself with additional food. Start slowly with moderate exercises and gradually increase your activity level. People who have not already accustomed their bodies to vigorous exercise are prone to various injuries. Consult your physician before you start jogging or heavy weight-lifting.

Table 16.1

Desirable Weights*
Men of Ages 25 and Over

Weight in Pounds According to Frame (in indoor Clothing)

Height (with shoes on) 1-inch heels Feet	Inches	Small Frame	Medium Frame	Large Frame
5	2	112—120	118—129	126—141
5	3	115—123	121—133	129—144
5	4	118—126	124—136	132—148
5	5	121—129	127—139	135—152
5	6	124—133	130—143	138—156
5	7	128—137	134—147	142—161
5	8	132—141	138—152	147—166
5	9	136—145	142—156	151—170
5	10	140—150	146—160	155—174
5	11	144—154	150—165	159—179
6	0	148—158	154—170	164—184
6	1	152—162	158—175	168—189
6	2	156—167	162—180	173—194
6	3	160—171	167—185	178—199
6	4	164—175	172—190	182—204

Women of Ages 25 and Over

For girls between 18 and 25, subtract 1 pound for each year under 25.

(with shoes on)
2-inch heels

4	10	92— 98	96—107	104—119
4	11	94—101	98—110	106—122
5	0	96—104	101—113	109—125
5	1	99—107	104—116	112—128
5	2	102—110	107—119	115—131
5	3	105—113	110—122	118—134
5	4	108—116	113—126	121—138
5	5	111—119	116—130	125—142
5	6	114—123	120—135	129—146
5	7	118—127	124—139	133—150
5	8	122—131	128—143	137—154
5	9	126—135	132—147	141—158
5	10	130—140	136—151	145—163
5	11	134—144	140—155	149—168
6	0	138—148	144—159	153—173

*New weight tables now in the process of being formulated will show that desirable weights for men and women today probably are higher than those in the tables above which were based on statistical studies made 25 years ago.

Q. How does exercise affect our metabolic rates and our appetite-control patterns?

A. Our metabolic rate is the total of calories needed to maintain normal body functions while in the resting state, combined with the energy expended in exercise or work. Exercise increases the metabolic rate. Exercise can help you to bring your calorie expenditure into balance with your appetite. Furthermore, moderate exercise has a tranquilizing effect; it helps relieve the tension that causes us to overeat. Exercise also helps tone the muscles that cause the sagging of the abdominal walls, which can occur after excessive weight loss.

Table 16.2

ACTIVITY	GROSS ENERGY COST-CAL. PER HOUR
A. Rest and Light Activity	50—200 per hour
Lying down or sleeping	80
Sitting	100
Driving an automobile	120
Standing	140
Domestic work	180
B. Moderate Activity	200—350 per hour
Bicycling (5½ mph)	210
Walking (2½ mph)	210
Gardening	220
Canoeing (2½ mph)	230
Golf	250
Lawn mowing (power mower)	250
Bowling	270
Lawn mowing (hand mower)	270
Fencing	300
Rowboating (2½ mph)	300
Swimming (¼ mph)	300
Walking (3¾ mph)	300
Badminton	350
Horseback riding (trotting)	350
Square dancing	350
Volleyball	350
Roller skating	350
C. Vigorous Activity	over 350 per hour
Table tennis	360
Ditch digging (hand shovel)	400
Ice skating (10 mph)	400
Wood chopping or sawing	400
Tennis	420
Water skiing	480
Hill climbing (100 ft. per hour)	490
Skiing (10 mph)	600
Squash and handball	600
Cycling (13 mph)	660
Scull rowing (race)	840
Running (10 mph)	900

Q. Can I lose weight with the aid of meditation?

A. Loss of appetite control is largely due to tension. Dieting increases tensions. A program of meditation to reduce tensions can be very beneficial for people on a diet. But meditation will not burn extra calories. You need exercise and diet restriction to lose weight. Meditation can help you develop a positive mental attitude that will help you stick to your plan.

Q. Should I skip meals to lose weight?

A. Skipping meals is not a desirable way to lose weight. One will usually overcompensate on the next meal because he will be hungrier than normal. Many fat people eat only one good meal a day. This is not a desirable habit. We can consume more calories and still lose as much weight when we stay with three meals per day. This spares us added stress and provides a better nutrient balance.

Q. How can I determine which of the many kinds of diets is the right one for me?

A. The selection of a proper regimen should always be done in consultation with your physician. Almost everyone has a medical reason to avoid some diets.

There are, however, some guidelines to help you select the diet and exercise program best suited for you. Unless you are huge, it is not likely that you can safely sustain a weight loss of more than three or four pounds per week. One or two pounds per week is all that one can expect to lose without extreme sacrifice. Any program that promises excessively rapid weight loss is unsound and possibly dangerous. Heavy losses during the first week of abrupt introduction of a diet are common. But these changes are temporary, due to shifts in body fluids, shrinkage of stomach contents, etc. On the other hand, some people fail to experience weight loss for several days after they start a new diet. Sometimes fat burned from the cells is temporarily replaced with water. Fluid retention can cause disappointment early in the program, just as excessive loss of body water can cause false hope.

Beware of diets that promise you can lose weight

without changing your eating habits, that you can eat anything you want. If you supply your body with more calories than it needs, it will store them as body fat. CALORIES DO COUNT. If you expect to lose weight, you must take in fewer calories than your body needs, and allow body fat to be burned to make up that difference.

Any healthful diet must fill the need for all essential nutrients except those calorie requirements that can be satisfied by the breakdown of body fat. You will continue to need the essential vitamins and minerals, the essential fatty acids, a small amount of fat for absorption of the fat-soluble vitamins, carbohydrates to support certain metabolic functions, and essential amino acids to maintain lean body mass.

Q. What about fasting and the liquid protein fasts? Are these safe for weight managment?

A. Fasting has been used with hospitalized patients for very large weight losses. But because no food is ingested, one can expect to lose some essential body tissue mass. Usually skeletal muscle is most affected. But the heart may also be weakened, and it is possible for fasting to cause endocrine imbalances such as low thyroid activity. Starvation edema (water retention through swelling of the tissues) is another threat. Fasting is safe only under expert medical supervision.

To eliminate the wasting of lean body mass and make it possible to fast outside of the hospital setting, the protein-sparing modified fast was conceived. Proteins of high nutritional quality proved useful in successful weight reduction. Then proteins of poor nutritional quality (predigested gelatin, a liquid protein sold under a variety of brand names) were introduced. Even though some modification of these solutions was accomplished by the addition of essential nutrients, it is doubtful that such products can avoid the loss of essential tissue mass, and ketosis is a potential hazard to anyone taking these proteins and using them as the sole source of nutrients.

Q. What is ketosis?

A. Ketosis is a state of high levels of ketones in the

body. Ketones are produced in the body from the combustion of fats in the absence of carbohydrates. High-protein-low-carbohydrate diets cause excretion of ketones in the urine. Ketosis supposedly decreases the appetite, but some individuals get headaches, nausea, and vomiting when on ketogenic diets. Ketones can compete with uric acid for excretion in the kidneys, and cause increased uric acid in the blood, which can lead to gout or kidney damage. People on ketogenic diets should have blood tests to monitor their uric-acid level. Ketogenic diets should be used only under close medical supervision.

Q. Why do many people regain weight so rapidly after they go off their diets?

A. Often weight loss, particularly if it is very rapid, is accomplished by only a loss of body fluids. Such weight returns rapidly when the old diet is reestablished or when fluids are replaced simply by drinking. Any program, for long-term success, must train the individual to change his eating and drinking habits. He must not go back to his old regimen. Sometimes this requires stressful changes in lifestyle. Reeducation of the appetite-control center requires long-term support. Cyclic loss and gain of weight is dangerous.

Q. Do I need a vitamin-mineral supplement while on a reducing diet?

A. It is very difficult to meet the RDA's without a supplement. The RDA's (Recommended Daily Allowances) are the amounts of each nutrient believed by the Food and Nutrition Board of the National Research Council to be nearly optimum for Americans who consume the typical diet. Haphazard weight-loss diets fail to achieve these goals.

Q. What about diet pills? How do they work, and are they safe?

A. The exact way appetite-suppressing drugs work is unknown. The original of this class of drugs was an amphetamine. People often become tolerant to the effects of the drugs and have to increase the dosage after a few weeks in order to get the same appetite control. This is a potentially dangerous practice. Amphetamines can cause a "psychosis" very similar to some of the very severe mental disorders. Diet pills deal with appetite alone, and it is still necessary to follow a proper diet in order to lose fat. A well-conceived weight-management program can control the craving for food without the use of pills.

Q. My doctor said my triglycerides are high. What does that mean?

A. *Triglycerides* is another name for the common form of fat. Too much fat in the blood suggests that you are consuming too much rich food. Reduced caloric intake, coupled with an exercise program, will usually result in normal blood lipids (fats).

Q. Does high cholesterol mean the same thing as high triglycerides?

A. Cholesterol is a waxy kind of lipid or fatty substance in the blood. High cholesterol in the blood is associated with increased risk of cardiovascular disease. In most cases, the remedy for high cholesterol is the same as for triglycerides: Decrease your calorie intake and watch your consumption of hard (saturated) animal fats. In a minority of cases, there is a genetic predisposition to high cholesterol. Although the genetic disorder is relatively rare, about one of five heart-attack victims has it. A family history of heart attacks at an early age (in the forties) is suggestive of this form of metabolic disorder. These cases must be handled by very rigid dietary rules. Such persons must limit their consumption of cholesterol-rich foods. Smoking is another cause of high cholesterol in the blood.

Q. How can I avoid gaining weight when I quit smoking?

A. The weight gain will usually be eight pounds or less. That is a small price to pay for the benefits to be gained by cessation of smoking. You can concentrate on your weight problem after you have stabilized your nonsmoking habits. It is better not to add the stresses of dieting to the stresses of a new nonsmoking program. Exercise, however, can help you to live with the stresses

169

of nonsmoking while, at the same time, moderating your weight gain by using up some of the excess calories you may consume when you first quit smoking.

Q. My doctor said I should eat bananas. Why?

A. Some of the medications for high blood pressure cause loss of potassium through the urine. Potassium is important for normal heart rhythm. Bananas are fairly rich in potassium, as is also true of many other fruits and vegetables.

Q. My doctor said I should decrease my salt intake. How do I do that?

A. The first step is to take your salt shaker off the table!! Do not add any salt to your food. The chemical name for salt is sodium chloride. Sodium can cause water retention and contribute to high blood pressure. If your foods taste too bland without salt, try flavoring them with some of the herbs and spices.

Q. Why is fiber important in weight management?

A. Fiber helps to fill you up without producing calories, and there is evidence that a high-fiber diet decreases the risk of cancer of the colon. The increased bulk helps speed up the flow of wastes through the colon so that there is less time for adverse action of bacteria that convert the bile salts to potential cancer-causing agents.

Q. If I don't drink milk, how should I compensate for the lack of calcium in my diet?

A. One ounce of hard cheese is approximately equivalent to one glass of milk in calcium content. Buttermilk and/or yogurt are often well tolerated by persons who can't drink milk. If you do not use one of these foods regularly, it becomes advisable to take calcium supplements. Calcium carbonate (oyster shells or dolomite) or calcium gluconate tablets are usually satisfactory forms of calcium. About 500 mg. of calcium per day is usually an adequate supplement for adults.

Q. I want to become a vegetarian, but my friends say I could get a protein deficiency. How important are the proteins?

A. Most Americans get more protein than they need.

Vegetables contain protein, but the vegetable proteins are not used as efficiently as are the animal proteins. We speak of the degree to which a given protein is digested and utilized by the body for building new tissues as a measure of its "biological value." The legumes (dried beans, lima beans, peas, peanuts) are relatively high in protein of fairly high biological value. Cereal proteins have low biological values, but when they are combined with milk or cheese, their biological values increase. The essential factors missing in cereal proteins are abundant in milk proteins. Most vegetarians include dairy products and eggs (high-quality "complete" animal proteins) in their diets. So they are not vegetarians in a strict sense, but "ovo-lacto" vegetarians. When no animal protein is consumed, there is danger of vitamin B_{12} deficiency. Much caution is needed when there are growing children in your family. They need lots of complete (high biological value) protein to build enzymes and hormones, muscles, and other tissues for growth.

Q. How can I manage my weight when I eat in restaurants almost every day?

A. Restaurants are famous for their rich sauces and desserts. Ask that the sauce be omitted from the entree, and don't feel that you have to eat everything on your plate. It's better to let it go to waste than to your *waist*! Avoid the two-martini lunch. Alcohol contains almost as many calories per gram as fat, and it is detrimental to the appetite-control center.

Q. How does the method of cooking affect the value of the food I eat?

A. Of foremost importance for people on a weight-management program is that the smallest possible amount of fat be added in the preparation of food. Roasting meat on a rack, for example, will allow the fat to drip away from the meat, cutting its caloric content tremendously. Vegetables (e.g., potatoes) and eggs should not be fried. The fat that adheres to them can double their caloric content. On a weight basis, fat is two and one quarter times as high in calories as carbohydrates and proteins.

171

In addition to changes in calories, one should keep in mind that cooking methods using the least amount of water will usually be best for the conservation of vitamins and minerals. "Waterless" cookery, baking, and steaming are recommended methods of cooking. Nonstick frying pans offer an improvement over conventional frying pans. A newer method of cooking utilizes microwave ovens. Microwave cookery conserves nutrients because it requires less water than conventional methods, and it does not require the addition of fat for heat transfer.

Q. How can I motivate myself to stick with my weight-management program?

A. Make a list of your strongest desires, regardless of whether you expect them to materialize and no matter how unattainable they look on paper. Carry the list with you, and add to it any new desires that occur to you. Then, by the process of elimination, decide what you want most. The things you do not truly want will make you drowsy or bored when you think about them. You'll find yourself going to the refrigerator for a snack or something to drink. The things you really want will make you forget about bodily comforts, big meals, or something to drink. When you concentrate on things you truly, deeply, desperately want, you will forget the clock, creature comforts, vacations, and the nonessentials of life. If you truly want something, your subconscious will furnish you with ample reasons and full power for achieving it. Watch your memory in connection with anything you think you want. If you keep forgetting dates, appointments, or tasks related to what you think you want, you don't really have the desire for it. When you have arrived at an awareness of just what you really, truly want most, you will find that you must make yourself more healthy and more attractive in order to achieve these goals. Keep your conscious mind on the things you really, truly want to accomplish, and your subconscious mind will guide you to the means for achieving them. And—don't forget!—professionals in several medical and paramedical disciplines (psychology, nutrition, physical therapy, etc.) are trained and experienced in guiding people such as yourself over (or around) the barriers you will encounter. Do not hesitate to ask for their assistance.

APPENDIX

For Health Professionals—Nutrition, Obesity, Dietary Fiber, Estrogens, and Preventive Aspects of Diabetes Mellitus: Human Leads to an Experimental Approach

Abstract

In this presentation I review the epidemiology, biochemistry, endocrinology, metabolism, and nutritional aspects of diabetes mellitus. Studies on the international variation of the incidence of diabetes show that it is associated with the amounts of fat, fiber, and sugar in the diet. More than 90 percent of diabetes in the United States is due to our Westernized diet, while only 8 percent is due to genetic factors. High-fat, low-fiber diets increase the metabolic activity of the intestinal microflora that metabolize biliary steroids into estrogens. High fat intake also causes obesity in susceptible persons. In obese men, excess body weight is significantly correlated with basal immuno-reactive insulin and urinary estrone production rates. This estrone is derived from extraglandular tissues. Furthermore, obese men are characterized by androgen-estrogen imbalance, but do not suffer feminization or other biological effects. Administration of estrogens to males caused changes in liver metabolism and androgen-estrogen imbalance, with feminization. In obese postmentopausal women, estrone is the principal estrogen derived from the extraglandular tissues, and it is correlated with excess body

174

weight. Weight loss reversed the androgen-estrogen imbalance in obese human subjects.

Bilateral electrical lesions to the ventromedial hypothalamus of experimental animals resulted in hyperphagia, obesity, and the female type of hepatic steroid metabolism. Vagotomy reversed the obesity, showing hypothalamic involvement with hunger, metabolism, and control of hormone levels. When neonatal male rats were given anti-androgens, feminization characterized by retention of estrogen in the hypothalamus occurred, as well as an increase in female-type estrogen-binding protein concentration in the hypothalamus, and female-type hepatic steroid metabolism. This suggests the posibility that hormonal imbalances and their consequences can be caused not genetically but by the total environment (including nutrition) of the pre- or neonatal animals.

Small increments of insulin suppress hepatic glucose output. Following glucose ingestion by normal subjects, more than 85 percent is retained in the splanchnic bed, whereas an increased proportion of ingested glucose load escapes hepatic uptake and enters the circulation in diabetics. Furthermore, fasting diabetics are characterized by increased gluconeogenesis and failure of intravenous glucose to inhibit hepatic glucose output.

Obese newborns of diabetic mothers have hyperinsulinemia. The incidence of diabetes in the offspring of diabetic mothers is 20 times the normal. Significant correlations were found between the newborns of deabetic mothers with birth weight greater than 4 kilograms, and obesity. If one can prevent hyperglycemia and overnutrition during pregnancy and pre- and postnatal life, prevention of diabetes seems possible. More than 75 percent of obese men have abnormal glucose tolerance tests. Over 75 percent of diabetics are obese. Estrogens are significantly elevated in diabetic men. The pituitary is an insulin-sensitive organ. Pituitary response to lutinizing hormone-releasing hormone in insulin-dependent diabetics is defective. Weight loss as well as high-fiber, low-fat diets reversed these findings.

Amelioration of the hyperglycemia appears responsible for the reversibility of the abnormalities seen in diabetics.

A hypothesis is presented on how elevated plasma estrogens reversibly block the estradiol receptors in the liver, pituitary, and hypothalamus, cause hyperplasia of the beta cells of the pancreas and deterioration of the glucose homeostasis leading to diabetes mellitus.

There are more than ten million adult-onset and one million juvenile onset diabetics in the United States. In this country and in other parts of the world the incidence of diabetes is increasing with the rise in the standard of living. Because adult-onset diabetes is potentially reversible, new lines of investigation are needed to find its cause, so that this disease can be prevented. In this report I review the international epidemiology of diabetes. I also discuss the roles played by diet, nutrition, enterohepatic circulation, intestinal microflora, steroid synthesis by gut bacteria, fecal steroids, obesity, sex, parity, the effects of maternal diabetes on offspring, and metabolic and endocrine interactions.

The relative contributions of heredity and environment to the incidence of a chronic disease can be assessed epidemiologically by studying the disease among migrants (i.e., genetically similar groups in different environments) and among members of different racial or ethnic groups in an identical environment. If the incidence is different in migrant populations, the causal factor must be associated with lifestyles that change with the migration, whether or not a genetic factor is involved. The diseases with a genetic component are very seldom race-related (1).* Genetic factors such as mutation, selection, gene flow, and drift do not occur in short time spans of five to twenty-five years. Therefore chronic diseases that change in frequency or manifestation are likely to have an environmental rather than genetic origin.

* Figures in parentheses refer to reference notes following this chapter.

Epidemiology—International Variation

A comparison of the death rate due to diabetes mellitus in different countries revealed a higher death rate in countries with a Western lifestyle, such as the United States and Germany, than in Asian or African countries. These differences were more pronounced in females than in males. A comparison of the percentage prevalences of diabetes mellitus in Africa (Rhodesia), Japan (3), and the United States (4) is illustrated in Figure 2.5. I estimated the contributions of heredity, environmental factors, and Westernized diet. In these estimations I used the prevalence of diabetes mellitus in Africa as a baseline for heredity (0.4 percent), environmental contribution (0.03 percent) as the difference between the prevalence of diabetes mellitus in Japan and Africa, and the Westernized dietary contribution (4.57 percent) as the difference between the prevalence of diabetes mellitus in the United States and Japan. These estimations indicated that only 8 percent of the diabetes mellitus in the United States is due to heredity, while 91.4 percent is due to Westernized diet.

Epidemiology—Migrant Studies

I made a survey of the literature on the incidence, prevalance, and death rates due to diabetes mellitus in (a) Jewish ethnic groups in Israel (7); (b) Japanese in Japan (8,9) and Hawaii; and (c) Indians in India (10) and in Natal (South Africa) (11), Trinidad (12), and Fiji (13). These investigations revealed a common association between high dietary fat and sugar intake and death rates for diabetes (14). Higher incidence and higher death rates were also related to decreased fiber intake (15) and increased fat and high suger intake (2,3,6,16-19).

Himsworth reported how diet (a) determined glucose tolerance, (b) influenced the disease prior to onset, and (c) affected the incidence of diabetes mellitus (20,21,22). Shifting of the diet from high-fat to low-fat intake resulted in a change in sensitivity of the individual to the insulin secreted by his own pancreas (20). The diet of the diabetics before the onset of the disease contained equal protein, less carbohydrate, and more fat than the diets of normal subjects. Himsworth suggested "that the habitual ingestion of a diet containing of diminished proportion of carbohydrate may cause progressive permanent impairment of glucose tolerance and insulin sensitivity so that in the course of time, diabetes mellitus results" (21). He further stated "that the ingestion of a relatively low carbohydrate diet is the factor determining the onset of diabetes mellitus in individuals with a predisposition to the disease, and that if a high-carbohydrate diet had been taken, a considerable portion of these individuals would not have developed diabetes" (22). There have also been reports of remission of diabetes when a low-fat diet was eaten (23,24). On the other hand, increased total caloric intake rather than high fat intake had been implicated as the most important dietary factor responsible for diabetes mellitus (3,25).

Bacterial toxins either exogenously consumed or endogenously produced (such as alloxan or streptozotocin) have been implicated as the cause of the progressive decrease of the beta cells in maturity-onset diabetes (26,29). Epidemiological data from Africa, Japan, and Western countries however, do not support these theories (2,3,25).

Ninety percent of high-fat-fed rats with alloxan-induced diabetes died, while only 40 percent of those on a low-fat diet died (30). Also, high fat consumption induced increased ketonuria in a genetic diabetic model (31) Pancreatic beta cells obtained from obese rats were more susceptible to a diabetogenic agent, strepto-zotocin, after they were fed high-fat diets than those from lean rats fed low-fat diets (32).

High-Fat Diet and Intestinal Microflora

Some researches have determined that intestinal bacteria can change dietary fats into diabetes-causing agents.

Feces from British and American subjects showed higher counts of *Bacteroides* and lower counts of *Enterococci* and other aerobic bacteria than the feces of Japanese, Indians, and Ugandans (33), in whom the incidence of diabetes mellitus is lower.

Feces of people consuming Westernized diets contained various subspecies of *Bacteroides fragilis* as dominant members of the fecal flora, besides large numbers of species of anaerobes and aerobic forms (34). Fecal specimens from people living in geographical locations with low incidence of diabetes mellitus had fewer *Bacteroides* and more *Enterococci* than those living in areas of higher incidence (33,35). High-meat consumption resulted in higher counts for total anaerobic microflora as well as *Bacteroides Bifidobacterium peptococcus* and *Lactobacillus,* compared with non-meat-diet consumption (36).

Feces from Americans and Europeans contained higher concentrations of steroids than those of Africans or Asians, and the steroids were more degraded (33) in the latter groups. The time taken for transit of ingested markers through the intestinal tract of Western peoples is approximately double that of African villagers' transit times, while the weight of stool passed daily is half that passed by the Africans. These contrasts have been attributed to the difference between the low-residue refined Westernized diet and the high-residue traditional diet of the less-developed countries (37).

Estrogens seem to play a direct role in the etiology of diabetes mellitus (38–48). It had been shown that intestinal microflora can produce estrogens from the co-

Ionic biliary steroids (49). The role played by estrogens could explain the higher incidence of diabetes mellitus in women on the Westernized diet.

These findings support the thesis that geographical variations in the incidence of diabetes mellitus could depend partly on differences in diet which result in altered composition and metabolic activity of the gut bacteria.

Intestinal Microflora and Migration of Populations

Americans have lower counts of *Clostridium perfringens* in their stools than do native Japanese (50). *Fusobacteria* was the most common type in the feces of Japanese residing in both Japan and the United States who ate primarily Japanese foods (51). Few or no *Fusobacteria* were found in the feces of Japanese-Americans who ate a chiefly Westernized diet (51). *Fusobacteria* were markedly decreased in the feces of newly arrived Japanese in the United States who ate a chiefly Westernized diet, while the counts of *Fusobacteria* did not change in the feces of those who continued to eat Japanese foods after they arrived in the United States. There was no significant difference in the *Bacteroides* count among these groups (51).

Extremely oxygen-sensitive anaerobes were more commonly recovered from the stools of subjects on the Japanese diet than from those on the Westernized diet (52). Higher counts for *S. faecalis var faecalis,* certain facultative and aerobic organisms, nonsporing anaerobic bacilli, and of certain *peptostreptococcus* species were present in feces of the subjects on the Japanese diet. Higher counts of *Bacteroides Bifidobacterium infantis*, and *Bifragilis* in the stools of subjects on the Westernized diet were confirmed (52).

Fecal Microbial Enzymes and Diet

The activities of intestinal bacterial enzymes are changed by diet (53,54). Giving subjects ampicillin

180

changed their intestinal bacteria and caused an increase in the excretion of fecal estrogens (55,56).

A shift in diet from grain to meat has resulted in a 1.5 to 2.0-fold increase in the activity of fecal beta-glucuronidase, azoreductase, and nitroreductase in rats. Continued feeding of meat diets (57) for twenty months resulted in a further increase in the activity of these enzymes in rats.

Giving human subjects fiber supplements did not cause a significant increase in fecal enzyme activities for beta-glucuronidase, azoreductase, or nitroreductase (57). A high-meat diet gave rise to singificant increases in fecal beta-glucuronidase compared to a nonmeat Westernized diet in human volunteers (58).

NAD- and NADP-dependent fecal $7=\alpha=$hydroxy-steroid dehydrogenases were also changed with different diets. Seventh Day Adventists (vegetarians) had lower fecal enzymes than did omnivorous control subjects (59). *Clostridium paraputrificum,* an organism isolated from feces of normal human subjects, was found to possess 3-oxo-5β-steroidΔ-4-dehydrogenase and 3-oxy-5β-steroidΔ-1-dehydrogenase activities (60). Aromatization (forming double bonds) of androst-4-ene-3, 17-dione was also demonstrated by this organism when this compound was converted to 17-methoxy-oestrien-1, 3, 5 (10)-3-OL (61). Four different mechanisms were proposed for the incorporation of double bonds in the steroid nucleus to give cyclopentaphenanthrene derivatives (62-64). Three out of the four reactions were shown to be carried out by *Clostridium paraputrificum.* It is of interest that several human microbial enzymes have been associated with the metabolism of bile acids and cholesterol into estrogens and other metabolites (64).

Fecal Steroids and Diet

Fecal production of estrone, estradiol, and a series of unidentified steroids with a phenolic ring A from 4-cholesterol-3-one was demonstrated, and bile acid with a phenolic ring A from 3-oxo-4-cholenic acid was produced (49). One of these compounds is a 17-substituted estrogen. The intestinal microbial synthesis of androstendione, cholestenone, and 3-oxo-chol-4en-24-oic acid was also established.

Low-fat intake decreased fecal acid steroids and neutral steroids (66). Chemically defined liquid low-fat diets promoted reduced excretion of both acid and neutral steroids (66).

When cholesterol is introduced into the colons of guinea pigs, it is metabolized to estradiol and appears later in the urine (67). People vary greatly in the amount of steroidal estrogens that are produced by their intestinal microflora (49). The quantities of these estrogens are much higher in people living on a Westernized diet than in those living on low-fat diets common in Africa, Asia, and South America. An 8 percent yield of 17-methoxy-estradiol from androstendione was produced by a culture of Clos. para. When volunteers ate Westernized diets, they excreted an average of 600 mg. a day of acid and neutral steroids (49). Their gut bacteria must aromatize only a small proportion of this substrate for its effect to be highly significant (49). When a bacterial culture obtained from the caecal contents of adult rats was incubated under nitrogen, estrone in amounts up to 42 percent of the concentration of estradiol was formed (68).

Lombardi et al. (69) have extensively investigated the metabolism of androgens and estrogens in human fecal microorganisms. Modification of androgens and estrogens were observed in incubations with mixed human fecal cultures, including both oxidative and reductive reactions (69). Reactions with high human fecal concentrations resulted in the products formed by reduction (69). Reactions with low concentrations in human feces resulted in the products formed by oxidation and by cleavage of conjugated steroids (69). Estrogen conjugated estrone 3-sulfate and estradiol-3-glucuronide were hydrolyzed to form estrone and estradiol, respectively. Metabolites of estrogens and androgens varied in human feces, depending on the concentration of feces and the availability of oxidizing agents such as phenazine methosulfate and menadione (69).

Biliary Excretion, Enterohepatic Circulation, and Detoxification Mechanisms

The nature of the hepatic conjugates will determine the ultimate fate of estrogens. The deconjugation of estradiol 3-sulfate by gut bacteria could cause the estradiol to be returned to the peripheral circulation and excreted later in urine, or directly excreted into bile. It could also be metabolized by gut bacteria. Most of it would undergo further metabolism and conjugation in the liver during enterohepatic circulation. The intestinal reabsorption of estriol and its conjugates is passive except for estriol 3-sulfate-16 α glucuronide, which is not readily absorbed because of its size. The latter conjugate is hydrolyzed by gut bacteria (70).

Estrone occurs mainly as the sulfate, estradiol as glucuronide, and estriol as the double conjugate 3-sulfate-16 α glucuronide. Estrone sulfate was better absorbed from the intestine than the free compounds (71). Up to 18 percent of the metabolites of estrone and estradiol are excreted in the feces. Because more than 50 percent of the metabolites are excreted in the bile of patients with biliary fistula, a greater part of the estrogen metabolites excreted into the bile is reabsorbed from the intestine and participates in enterohepatic circulation (71).

In a preliminary communication, it was recently reported that vegetarian women excreted 2 to 3 times more estrogen in their feces than did omnivorous ones, and that omnivorous women had about 50 percent higher mean plasma level of unconjugated estrone and estradiol than vegetarians (72). Estriol-3-glucuronide, a compound that is formed upon reabsorption of free estriol from the intestine was found in lower concentrations in the urine of vegetarian women. These data suggested that in vegetarians a great amount of the biliary estrogens escaped reabsorption and are excreted with the feces (72). The differences in the estrogen metabolism may explain why fewer vegetarians get diabetes.

High-Fiber Diets and Biliary Steroids

Increasing dietary fat intake also increased the fecal bile acid concentration in human subjects (73). Increasing the fiber content of the diet did the opposite. Bile acids undergo enterohepatic circulation in the intestine. There was active transport mechanism for their recovery from the gut lumen. Under "normal" physiological conditions, more than 98 percent of the bile acids were recovered. If this ability is reduced from 98 percent to 97 percent, there would be a 50 percent increase in the fecal loss of bile acids. Because the intestinal microflora can be changed by diet, the deconjugated products could alter the biological activity, toxicity, excretion, and reabsorption of many endogenous and exogenous compounds, such as acid and neutral steroids, ammonia and certain amides, major products of urea and protein degradation and tryptophane metabolites. Diet may also control the liver's secretory and functional ability (74) to yield potentially harmful metabolites that are subsequently split and released by gut bacteria.

The reported long-term beneficial effects of high-carbohydrate, high-fiber diets (75) could be related to the low-fat (27 percent of total calories) content of the diets. The lack of fat decreases the metabolic activity of the intestinal microflora and consequently decreases the production of bile acids and sex hormones. It was indeed interesting that McCarroll et al. (76) found non-hormonal factors to cause improvement of diabetes when the diabetics were fed high-fiber diets.

High-Fat Diet and Obesity

The endocrine and metabolic effects induced by high fat intake and short-term obesity in normal individuals are well characterized (77, 78).

Basal immunoreactive insulin is highly correlated with the percentage of body fat of animals. In all animals studied, leaner animals displayed lower fasting imunoreactive insulin values and fatter animals have higher ones (79). Obesity and both basal (80) and stimulated immunoreactive insulin levels are highly correlated in animals, including man (81, 82). Furthermore, hyperinsulinemia characteristic of obesity is a result of dietary factors and is not exclusively a consequence of the insulin antagonism associated with obesity (82-85).

Very recently, Nagulesparan et al. (86) were able to differentiate two reasons for the increased insulin resistance to glucose disposal in glucose-intolerant subjects: (1) obesity and (3) "other unknown factors." These unknown factors could arise from the diet-realted intestinal synthesis of estrogens.

Obesity and Estrogens in Men

While in women gross obesity has been associated with increased conversion of circulating androgens to estrogens (87), obesity in men has been associated with low serum testosterone levels (88-90), as well as low serum sex hormone binding globulin (SHBG) levels (88-91). Obesity in men has also been associated with marked elevation of plasma estrone, plasma estradiol, and urinary excretion (91-93). These estrogens are made not only by the intestinal microflora but by extraglandular tissues as well (49, 61-64, 94-98). Also in men obesity has been associated with normal serum gonadotropins (LH, FSH) (92, 93), and normal testosterone responses to clomiphene citrate, indicating that the hypothalamic-pituitary-Leydig cell axes are intact (91). To the degree that a man is above ideal body weight, his metabolic clearance rates (MCR) of testosterone and peripheral conversion of testosterone to estradiol and androstenedione to estrone are all increased (91, 92). Weight loss was accompanied by a progressive decline in estrone from 2½ normal to midnormal (p<0.001). At 8 weeks, there was significant reduction in androstenedione, while testosterone increased. In contrast, gonadotrophins remained unchanged. With weight loss, the abnormal hormonal state, including SHBG levels, returned to normal over several weeks, and estrone decreased 67 percent (93,99). Androstenedione was reduced only 34 percent, suggesting that decreased peripheral aromatization of androstenedione was another beneficial effect of weight loss.

Although obese men exhibited increased blood levels and production rates of estrogens, there were no signs of feminization. SHBG levels and basal gonadotrophin levels were normal. The apparent lack of biological effect is probably the reason hormonal causes for diabetes were not investigated sooner. However, 50 to 70 percent of diabetic men are impotent.

Obesity and Estrogens in Postmenopausal and Young Women

The metabolic clearance rate of estrogens in young women is about four times that in postmenopausal women (100). The prinicpal estrogen formed in postmenopausal women is estrone and is derived from the fat tissue by aromatization of plasma androstenedione (101,102), and enters the blood unaltered (103). Furthermore, estrogens are often given to postmenopausal women as hormone replacement therapy (104). The amount of plasma androstenedione converted to estrone is significantly correlated with total body weight and with excess body weight in young women(105). Altered hepatic metabolism of estrogens is also reported (106). When the diabetes death rate for postmenopausal women in different countries was compared, it was found that those consuming a diet low in fat and sugar had low death rates, while those consuming a diet high in these nutrients had a high rate (6). Obesity is common in postmenopausal women. It is tempting to speculate that obesity induces a reversible excess of estrogens that help cause diabetes. Indeed, Joslin et al. postulated

186

that menopause is one of the risk factors of diabetes mellitus (107).

Estrogens and Carbohydrate Metabolism

Giving estrogens to partially depancreatized, nonglucosuric rats fed on high-fat diets produced severe glucosuria and hyperglycemia (41). In another study nonpregnant rats were given doses of estradiol for three weeks. Both basal islet secretion and secretion during a thirty-minute intravenous glucose tolerance test were significantly increased (39).

The administration of ethinyl estradiol and dimethisterone to nonobese women for twenty-one days did not change either oral or intravenous glucose tolerance, but did cause hyperinsulinism and a threefold increase in human growth hormone (40).

Some of the effects of giving oral contraceptives containing synthetic estrogens and progesterones were as follows: (a) altered liver function; (b) excess circulating cortisol; (c) excess circulating growth hormone; (d) binding to insulin and inactivation of the biologic activity; (e) up to 39 percent of women receiving oral contraceptives had abnormal oral glucose tolerance test (OGTT); and (f) reversibility of metabolic changes if they are detected early and oral contraceptives are discontinued (42–46,48). Also, many women who were on birth control pills had decreased oral glucose tolerance during pregnancy and later became permanently diabetic (48).

Ventromedial Hypothalamic Obesity

Bilateral electrolytic lesions of the ventromedial hypothalamus (VMH) of male albino rats resulted in hyperphagia, weight gain, and obesity (108,109). Subdiaphragmatic vagotomy reversed the weight gain and the obesity in these animals (109). When rats with hypothalamic lesions were fed a high-fat diet, vagotomy did not reverse the obesity. When genetically obese Zucker rats were used for the same experiment, vagotomy did not reverse their obesity either. The current concepts of ventrolateral hypothalamic (VLH) regulation of the feeding center (insulin secretion and increased feeding) and VMH control of the satiety center have been recently reviewed (79).

Estrogen Receptors and Hypothalamus

Neonatal male rats treated with an antiandrogen (cyproterone) demonstrated several biological effects of "feminization," such as cyclic output of gonadotropins and female-type sex steroid (estradiol) retention by the anterior and the rostral middle hypothalamus. These two hypothalamic regions and the VMH are known to distinguish sex differences toward testosterone and estradiol (111), and are known to possess important sites of estradiol binding proteins in the adult female (112–115). Also, it is known that estrogen receptors in the rat hypothalamus develop during growth (116, 117).

"Feminization" and Hepatic Steroid Metabolites in the Male

Sex differences in the hepatic metabolism of androgens and estrogens are well known in the rat (118). Prenatal "feminization" of the male rat has induced changes in the enzyme activities of the microsomal metabolism of the liver in the direction characteristic of the female rats (119).

Following induction of an electrothermic lesion in the median eminence of the hypothalamus of the male rat, the hepatic steriod metabolism in the male was "feminized," indicating that the release of the pituitary feminizing factor is controlled by means of a release-inhibiting factor from the hypothalamus (120). Also, estradiol administration to castrated adult male rats resulted in a marked shifting of conjugation and oxido-reduction activities of the liver cell toward that of the female pattern (121). There is evidence to suggest that sex-differentiated hepatic steroid metabolism may occur in humans. The biological significance of sex differences in hepatic steriod metabolism is not clear, but it has been suggested that it is involved in protecting the organism from unwanted steriods (122).

Sex, Parity, and Diabetes

Fitzgerald et al. (123) found that the onset of diabetes is more common in men than in women before the age of forty. After that age, as the incidence in both sexes increases, more women than men were affected. The incidence of diabetes mellitus increases with parity. Compared with childless women, mothers of three are twice as likely to get diabetes, and women with six or more children are six times as likely to contract the disease (123).

Obesity and Diabetes in Mothers and Offspring

Obese newborns and the children of diabetic mothers both usually have too much insulin in their blood (124). That condition might be caused by an increased transplacental transfer of nutrients. The offspring of diabetic mothers have twenty times the incidence of diabetes than is found in the general population (124). Children of diabetic mothers demonstrated a paradoxical growth hormone secretion. Children born in periods with a high food supply displayed a significantly increased incidence of diabetes mellitus over subjects born in periods of food shortage (124,125). The majority of cases of familial diabetes have been observed on the maternal side(124). When the mothers were diabetic, newborns with a birth weight of more than 4000 gm. showed a significantly increased incidence of overweight at school age (124).

Even in nondiabetic mothers, increased weight of their offspring at birth was highly correlated with overweight at age 15 (124,125). Similarly, a highly significant positive corellation existed between the weight gain during the first three months of postnatal life and body weight at 15 years of age. Also, birth weights of greater than 4000 gm. are known to be significantly correllated with the development of diabetes later in life (124, 125).

Prenatal environment (88) plays an important role in causing diabetes mellitus. A well-controlled diabetic pregnant mother who does not overfeed herself or her baby can possibly prevent obesity and diabetes mellitus in the child (124,125).

Obesity, Estrogens, and Glucose Intolerance and Diabetes Mellitus

Obesity was even chosen as the central theme of a recent text on diabetes mellitus (3). An epidemic of obesity has also recently been reported in an American Indian population known to be highly susceptible to diabetes (126). Seventy-five percent of obese men have abnormal OGTTs (92,127). The diabetic's inability to maintain glucose homeostasis is often causally related to the onset and degree of obesity (128). Seventy-five percent of diabetics are obese (107). Plasma estradiol was significantly elevated in latent diabetic boys ($p \angle 0.05$) (129) and elevated in insulin-treated diabetic men (130). Diabetic women often have significant and striking differences in their rates of uriniary excretion of steroids (131). The findings, which were based on dexamethazone-suppression tests, synthetic beta-1,24-corticotropin stimulation tests, and intravenous stimulation by high doses of chorionic gonadotropin, suggested intact pituitary-adrenal Leydig cell axes (129). However, the pituitary is an insulin-sensitive organ (132,133). Furthermore, insulin dependent diabetics have defective pituitary responsiveness to lutinizing hormone-releasing hormone (134). The insulin response to oral glucose is absent, but a distinct response of glucagon to arginine is present in diabetic subjects

(135). Weight loss restored the normal fasting plasma glucose levels in diabetic subjects (135). The response of serum insulin levels to glucose in diabetic subjects increased significantly after weight loss, compared to initial values (p $\angle$ 0.001), but there was no change in glucagon response to arginine (135). Fasting plasma glucagon levels were reduced, and the degree of glucagon suppression in response to glucose in diabetic subjects, while enhanced (p $<$ 0.05), remained impaired compared to responses in control subjects (p $\angle$ .05). Mononuclear cell-insulin binding increased after weight loss (p $\angle$ 0.05) but was similar in both diabetics and control groups—both before and after weight loss. These results indicate that diabetics lose their glucose-induced insulin-secretory capacity, but amelioration of the hyperglycemia seems to reverse the loss. Diminished cellular receptor binding in obese subjects, by increasing resistance to the action of insulin, aggravated hyperglycemia and thereby contributed to the loss of beta-cell sensitivity to glucose (135). Similar to the benefits of weight reduction, benefit was also achieved with high-fiber, low-fat diets (136–139). High-fiber diets modified the composition of the intestinal micorflora (140).

Diabetes Mellitus-Glucose Homeostasis by the Liver and Splanchnic Glucose Balance after Glucose Ingestion

It is well known that the liver is a major site of insulin action in the regulation of glucose homeostasis (141). In normal subjects, small increments in insulin suppress hepatic glucose output without increasing peripheral glucose utilization (142). Following glucose ingestion, the major portion is retained within the splanchnic bed, while only 15 percent is available for disposal by peripheral tissues (141). In the insulin-deficient diabetic, both increased gluconeogenesis in the fasting state and the failure of intravenous glucose to inhibit hepatic glucose output have been demonstrated (143). Furthermore, a greater proportion of an ingested glucose load escapes hepatic uptake and enters the systemic circulation in diabetics than it does in normal subjects (144). Also, both portal and central hepatic cells of the diabetic liver contained significantly higher concentrations of pyridine-nucleotides (p<00.001) than those of normal livers (145).

Interaction Between Female Sex Hormones and Liver

Giving estrogens to humans causes decreased clearance of bilirubin from the plasma and intrahepatic cholestasis with necrosis of the liver cells but no inflammation (146). All values of bromsulfalein retention, alkaline phosphatase, and transaminase activity increased (146). Estrogens have been implicated as causing decreased secretion of substances into the bile and increased back diffusion from the bile into the blood. Biliary excretion of estrogens is a subject of a recent review (147). Hormonal imbalance and consequent "feminization" have been reported in patients with hepatic cirrhosis (148,149) and alcoholic liver disease. Serum total and free estradiol levels were significantly higher in men with cirrhosis than in normal men (148). In cirrhosis patients, the serum lutinizing hormone concentration was elevated, but follicle-stimulating hormone levels were normal (148). Similar findings were reported for men with fatty liver and chronic hepatitis (150). These elevated estrogens were derived from the peripheral conversion of androgens (151). Primary hypothalamic-pituitary suppression was postulated in alcoholic liver disease (152). Indeed, a recent report differentiated the effect of alcohol from that of cirrhosis and presented evidence supporting the direct effect of alcohol on hypothalamic-pituitary-gonadal-axis (153).

Postulated Hypothesis

More than 90 percent of the adult-onset diabetes in the Untied States is caused by the consumption of a Wes-

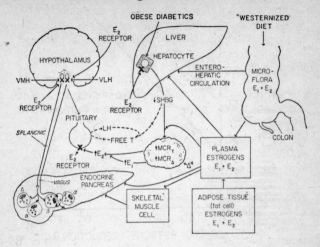

ternized diet, characterized by high fat and sugar content and low fiber content. This diet induces: (a) stepped-up conversion of bile acids to estrogens in the intestinal tract and (b) obesity, which often precedes diabetes. Also, the adipose tissue of the obese diabetic synthesizes a reversible excess of estrogens, which results in both a reversible estrogen-androgen imbalance and an excess of urinary estrogens in proportion to the percentage of excess body weight.

This hormonal imbalance shows specific biological effects: (a) no elevation in circulating sex hormone-binding globulin levels, (b) no suppression of pituitary gonadotropins, (c) defective hypothalamic gonadotropin-releasing-hormone production, (d) no sex signs of "feminization," and (e) altered hepatic steroid and carbohydrate metabolism.

Elevated plasma estrone either blocks or blunts the estradiol receptors in the liver, pituitary, and hypothalamus. The skeletal muscle and fat cells are desensitized to insulin action through the production of excess

Figure A.2

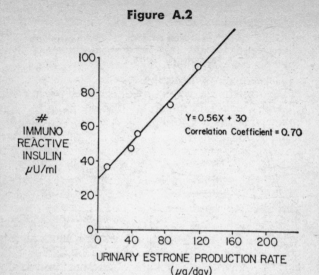

Y = 0.56X + 30
Correlation Coefficient = 0.70

\# IMMUNO REACTIVE INSULIN μU/ml

URINARY ESTRONE PRODUCTION RATE (μg/day)

growth hormone and glucocorticoids that result in hyperplasia of the beta cells. The blocking of estradiol receptors within the hepatocyte leads to unopposed androgen action, and, hence, sex-hormone-binding globulin production is not elevated. A decrease in sex-hormone-binding globulin results in an increase in the metabolic clearance rate (MCR) of testosterone and androstenedione because their clearances are inversely proportional to this binding protein. Gondaotropin levels remain normal because increased estrone production resulting from androgen metabolism blocks the estradiol receptors in the pituitary and hypothalamus. This could explain why, in diabetes, alterations in clearance and metabolism of androgens as well as elevated estrone production are noted. As a consequence, individuals with diabetes mellitus will develop (a) an excess of fasting insulin in proportion to urinary estrone excretion, (b) a decreased binding of insulin cellular receptors, and (c) an altered hepatic carbohydrate metabolism. The excess sugar intake present in the

194

Westernized diet thus escapes hepatic uptake, enters the systemic circulation, and causes the glucose intolerance characteristic of diabetes mellitus. Fortunately, these conditions are reversible.

The hyperglycemia and overnutrition characteristic of the Westernized diet may cause prenatal obesity with hyperinsulinemia in infants of diabetic mothers. This could make these infants more susceptible to diabetes mellitus. Fortunately, weight reduction with high-fiber, low-fat, low-sugar diets reverse these effects. So it seems that genuine preventive therapy, the highest aim in medicine, can be achieved by correcting the prenatal internal environment during the critical developmental periods of the neuroendocrine systems.

Animal models for diabetes and all types of obesity are available. By raising some of these animal models under appropriate germ-free conditions, we should be able to isolate the contribution of intestinal microbially synthesized estrogens. I also suggest in vitro experiments employing the liver, pituitary, or hypothalamus from these animal models. From these we might some day understand the mechanism of the blocking of the estradiol receptors, and progress toward the development of drugs that may overcome the harmful side effects of diabetes mellitus.

FIGURE LEGENDS

A.1. A hypothesis to explain the effect of diabetes mellitus on androgen-estrogen metabolism in man. $E_2=$ estradiol, $E_1=$ estrone, SHBG-sex-hormone-binding globulin, $MCR_r=$ metabolic clearance rate of testosterone, $MCR\Delta=$ metabolic clearance rate of androstenedione. LH= lutinizing hormone, T= testosterone, VMH = Ventro-medial hypothalamus, VLH = ventro-lateral hypothalamus, $\beta=\beta$ cells, $\alpha=\alpha$ cells, $\Delta=\Delta$ cells of the islets of Langerhans.

A.2. Correlation between the urinary estrone production and basal immunoreactive insulin in obese men (72,77).

References for Appendix

1. Damon, A. Race, ethnic group, and disease. *Social Biol.* 16:69, 1969.
2. *World Health Statistics*, Vital statistics and causes of death. Vol. I. 1973.
3. West, K.M. Epidemiology of diabetes and its vascular complications. New York: Elsevier, 1978.
4. *Report of the National Commission on Diabetes*, Dept. Health, Education and Welfare Publication, (N.I.H. No. 76–1022) 3:35, 1975.
5. Wynder, E.L. and G.B. Gori. Contribution of the environment to cancer incidence: An epidemiologic exercise. *J. Natl. Cancer Inst.* 58:825, 1977.
6. Higginson, J. Present trends in cancer epidemiology. *Proc. Can. Cancer Conf.* 8:40, 1969.
7. Medalie, J.H., J.B. Herman, V. Goldbourt and C.M. Papier. Variations in incidence of diabetes among 10,000 adult Israeli males and the factors related to their development. In *Advances in Metabolic Disorders,* edited by M. Miller and P.H. Bennett. New York: Academic Press, 1978, Vol. 9, p. 94.
8. Kawate, R., M. Miyanishi, M. Yamakido and Y. Nishimoto. Preliminary studies of the prevalence and mortality of diabetes mellitus in Japanese in Japan and on the island of Hawaii. In *Advances in Metabolic Disorders,* edited by M. Miller and P.H. Bennett. New York: Academic Press, 1978, Vol. 9, p. 201.
9. Kawate, R., M. Yamakido, Y. Nishimoto, P.H. Bennett, R.F. Hamman and W.C. Knowler. Diabetes mellitus and its vascular complications in Japanese migrants on the island of Hawaii. *Diabetes Care,* 2:161, 1979.
10. Gupta, O.P., M.H. Joshi and S.K. Dave. Prevalence of diabetes in India. In *Advances in Metabolic Disorders,* edited by M. Miller and P.H. Bennett. New York: Academic Press, 1978, Vol. 9, p. 147.
11. Jackson, W.P.U. Epidemiology of diabetes in South Africa. In *Advances in Metabolic Disorders*, edited by M.

Miller and P.H. Bennett. New York: Academic Press, 1978, Vol. 9, p. 112.

12. Poon-King, T., M.V. Henry and F. Rampersad. Prevalence and natural history of diabetes in Trinidad. *Lancet* i:155, 1968.

13. Cassidy, J.T. Diabetes in Fiji. *New Zealand Med. J.* 66:167, 1967.

14. *Provisional Food Balanced Sheets*, Food and Agriculture Organization, United Nations, 1972–74.

15. Trowell, H.C. The development of the concept of dietary fiber in human nutrition. *Am. J. Clin. Nutr.* 31:S3, 1978.

16. Adamson, L.F. Serum Cholesterol concentrations of various ethnic groups in Hawaii. *J. Nutr.* 60:27, 1971.

17. Antonis, A. and I. Berohn. The influence of diet on fecal lipids in South Africa and white and Bantu prisoners. *Am. J. Clin. Nutr.* 11:142, 1962.

18. Weinsier, R.L., A. Seeman, M.G. Herrera, J.P. Assal, J.S. Soeldner and R.E. Gleason. High- and low-carbohydrate diets in diabetes mellitus. Study of effects on diabetic control, insulin secretion, and blood lipids. *Ann. Int. Med.* 80:332, 1974.

19. Yudkin, J. Dietary fat and dietary sugar in relation to Ischaemic heart disease and diabetes. *Lancet* ii:4, 1964.

20. Himsworth, H.P. The dietetic factor determining the glucose tolerance and sensitivity to insulin of healthy men. *Clin. Sci.* 2:67, 1935.

21. Himsworth, H.P. and E.M. Marshall. The diet of diabetics prior to the onset of the disease. *Clin. Sci.* 2:95, 1935.

22. Himsworth, H.P. Diet and the incidence of diabetes mellitus. *Clin. Sci.* 2:117, 1935.

23. Harwood, R. Severe diabetes with remission. Report of a case and review of the literature. *N. Eng. J. Med.* 257:257, 1957.

24. Genuth, S.M. Effects of prolonged fasting on insulin secretion. *Diabetes* 15:798, 1966.

25. Renold, A.E., D.H. Mintz, W.A. Muller and G.F. Cahill, Jr. Diabetes mellitus. In *The Metabolic Basis of Inherited Disease,* edited by J.B. Stanbury, J.B. Wyngaarden, and D.S. Fredrickson. New York: McGraw-Hill, 1978, p. 80.

26. Issenberg, P. Nitrite, nitrosamines and cancer. *Fed. Proc.* 35:1322, 1976.

27. Berne, C., R. Gunnersson, C. Hellerstrom and E. Wilander. Diabetogenic nitrosoamines. *Lancet* i:173, 1974.

28. Wilander, E. Streptozotocin—diabetes in the Chinese hamster. Volumetric quantitation of the pancreatic islets and inhibition of diabetes with nicotinamide. *Horm. Metab. Res.* 7:15, 1975.

29. Wilander, E. and R. Gunnarsson. Diabetogenic effects of

N-nitrosomethyl urea in the Chinese hamster. *Acta Path. Microbiol. Scand. Sect.* A-83:206, 1975.

30. Houssay, B.A. and C. Martinez. Experimental diabetes and diet. *Science* 105:548, 1947.

31. Grodsky, G.M., B.J. Frankel, J.E. Gerich, and G.C. Gerritsen. The diabetic Chinese hamster: In vitro insulin and glucagon release. The chemical diabetic; and the effect of diet on ketonemia. *Diabetologia* 10:521, 1974.

32. Inoue. S. and A.G. Bray. Sensitivity of B-cells to streptozotocin in lean and obese rats. *Horm. Metab. Res.* 10:273, 1978.

33. Hill, M.J., J.S. Crowther, B.S. Drasar, G. Hawksworth, V. Aries and R.E.O. Williams. Bacteria and etiology of cancer of large bowel. *Lancet* i:95, 1971.

34. Atterbery, H.R., V.L. Sutter and S.M. Finegold. Normal human intestinal flora. In *Anaerobic Bacteria—Role in Disease*, edited by A. Balows, R.M. Dettan, V.R. Dowell, Jr., L.B. Guze. Springfield, Illinois: Charles C. Thomas, 1974, p. 81.

35. Hill, M.J. and B.S. Drasar Bacteria and the etiology of cancer of the large intestine. In *Anaerobic Bacteria—Role in Disease*, edited by A. Balows, R.M. Dattan, V.R. Dowell, Jr., L.B. Guze. Springfield, Illinois: Charles C. Thomas, 1974, p. 119.

36. Reddy, B.S., J.H. Weisburger and E.L. Wynder. Effects of high risk and low risk diets on colon carcinogenesis on fecal microflora and steroids in man. *J. Nutr.* 105:878, 1975.

37. Burkitt, D.P., A.R.P. Walker and N.S. Painter. Effect of dietary fiber on stools and transit-times, and its role in the causation of disease. *Lancet* ii:1408, 1972.

38. Adams, P.W. and N.W. Oakley. Oral contraceptives and carbohydrate metabolism. *Clinic End. Metab.* 1:697, 1972.

39. Costrini, N.V. and V. Kalkhuff. Relative effects of pregnancy, estradiol, and progesterone on plasma insulin and pancreatic islet insulin secretion. *J. Clin. Invest.* 50:992, 1971.

40. Yen, S.S.C. and P. Vela. Effects of contraceptive steroid on carbohydrate metabolism. *J. Clin. Endocrinol.* 28:1564, 1968.

41. Ingle, D.T. Diabetogenic effect of stilbestrol in force-fed normal and partially depancreatized rats. *Endocrinol.* 29:838, 1941.

42. Spellacy, W.N. Progestogen and estrogen effects on carbohydrate metabolism. In *Uterine Contraction—Side Effects of Steroidal Contraceptives*, edited by J.B. Josinovich. New York: John Wiley, 1973, p. 327.

43. Kalkhoff, R.K. Effects of oral contraceptive agents on

carbohydrate metabolism. *J. Steroid Biochem.* 6:949, 1975.

44. Spellacy, W.N., W.C. Buhi and S.A. Birk. Norgestrel and carbohydrate-lipid metabolism: glucose, insulin and triglyceride changes during six months time of use. *Contraception* 9:615, 1974.

45. Javier, Z., H. Gershberg and M. Hulse. Ovulatory suppressants, estrogens and carbohydrate metabolism. *Metabolism* 17:443, 1968.

46. Pyorala, K., T. Pyorala and V. Lampinen. Oral contraceptive treatment and intravenous glucose tolerance. *Lancet* ii:776, 1967.

47. Malaisse, W.J. Hormonal and environmental modification of islet activity. In *Handbook of Physiology, Endocrinology I*, edited by D.F. Steiner. Washington:American Physiological Society, 1972, p. 237.

48. Gershberg, H., Z. Javier and M. Hulse. Glucose tolerance in women receiving an ovulatory suppressant. *Diabetes* 13:378, 1964.

49. Hill, M.J., P. Goddard and R.E.O. Williams. Gut bacteria and etiology of cancer of the breast. *Lancet* ii:472, 1971.

50. Akama, K. and S. Otani. Clostridium perfringens as the flora in the intestine of healthy persons. *Jap. J. Med. Sci. Biol.* 23:161, 1970.

51. Ueno,, P.T. Sugihara, K.S. Bricknell, H.R. Attebery, V.L. Sutter and S.M. Finegold. Comparison of characteristics of gram-negative anaerobic bacilli isolated from feces of individuals in Japan and the United States. In *Anaerobic Bacteria—Role in Disease*, edited by A. Balows, R.M. Dettan, V.R. Dowell, Jr., L.B. Guze. Springfield, Illinois: Charles C. Thomas, 1974, p. 135.

52. Finegold, S.M., H.R. Attebery and V.L. Sotter. Effect of diet on human fecal flora: Comparison of Japanese and American diets. *Am. J. Clin. Nutr.* 27:1456, 1974.

53. Reddy, B.S. and E.L. Wynder. Large bowel carcinogenesis: Fecal constituents of populations with diverse incidence rates of colonic cancer. *J. Natl. Cancer Inst.* 50:1437, 1973.

54. Goldin, B.R. and S.L. Gorbach. The relationship between diet and rat fecal bacterial enzymes implicated in colon cancer. *J. Natl. Cancer Inst.* 57:371, 1976.

55. Adlercreutz, H., F. Martin, M. Pulkkinen, H. Dencker, V. Rimer, N.O. Sjoberg and M.J. Tikkanen Intestinal metabolism of estrogens. *J. Clin. Endocrinol. Metab.* 43:497, 1976.

56. Martin, F., J. Pellonen, T. Lautikainen, M. Pulkkinen and H. Adlercreutz. Excretion of progesterone metabolites and estriol in feces from pregnant women during amphicillin administration. *J. Steroid Biochem.* 6:1339, 1975.

57. Goldin, B., J. Dwyer, S.L. Gorback, W. Gordon and L. Swenson. Influence of diet and age on fecal bacterial enzymes. *Am. J. Clin. Nutr.* 31:S136, 1978.

58. Reddy, B.S., J.H. Weisburger and E.L. Wynder. Fecal bacterial B-glucoronidase: control by diet. *Science* 183:416, 1974.

59. Macdonald, I.A., G.R. Webb and D.E. Mahoney. Fecal hydroxysteroid dehydrogenase activities in vegetarian Seventh-Day Adventists, control subjects and bowel cancer patients. *Am. J. Clin. Nutr.* 31:S233, 1978.

60. Aries, V.C., P. Goddard and M.J. Hill. Degradation of steroids by intestinal bacteria III. 3-oxo-5B-steroid Δ^4-dehydrogenase. *Biochem. Biophys. Acta* 248:482, 1971.

61. Goddard, P. and M.J. Hill. Aromatization of androst-4-ene-3, 17-dione by human intestinal bacteria. *Biochem. J.* 124: 73P, 1971.

62. Goddard, P. and M.J. Hill. Degradation of steroids by intestinal bacteria. IV. The aromatization of ring A. *Biochem. Biophys. Acta* 280:336, 1972.

63. Goddard, P. and M.J. Hill. The degradation of the steroid nucleus by human gut bacteria. *Trans. Biochem. Soc.* 1:1113, 1973.

64. Hill, M.J. The role of colon anaerobes in the metabolism of bile acids and steroids and its relation to colon cancer. *Cancer* 36:2387, 1975.

65. Hill, M.J. The effect of some factors on the faecal concentration of acid steroids, neutral steroids and urobilins. *J. Path.* 104:239, 1971.

66. Crowther, J.S., B.S. Drasar, P. Goddard, M.J., Hill and K. Johnson. The effect of chemically defined diet of the fecal flora and fecal steroid concentration. *Gut* 14:790, 1973.

67. Goddard, P. and M.J. Hill. The in vivo metabolism of cholesterol by gut bacteria in the rat and guinea-pig. *J. Steroid. Biochem.* 5:569, 1974.

68. Amland, M.D. and K.F. Stoa. Metabolism of oestradiol-17β by intestinal bacteria in rats. *Horm. Res.* 6:366, 1975.

69. Lombardi, P., B. Goldin, E. Boutin and S.L. Gorback. Metabolism of androgens and estrogens by human fecal micro-organisms. *J. Steroid Biochem.* 9:795, 1978.

70. Taylor, W. The excretion of steroid metabolites in bile and feces. *Vit. Horm.* 29:201, 1971.

71. Latikainen, T. Quantitative studies on the excretion of glucoronide and mono- and disulphate conjugates of neutral steroids in human bile. *Ann. Clin. Res.* 2:338, 1970.

72. Goldin, B.R., H. Adlercreutz, J.T. Dwyer, L. Swenson, J.H. Warram and S.L. Gorbach. The effect of diet on excretion of estrogens in pre- and postmenopausal

women. Paper presented during fat and cancer workshop in Bethesda. Maryland. 1979.

73. Antonis, A. and I. Berohn. The influence of diet on fecal lipids in South African white and Bantu prisoners. *Am. J. Clin Nutr.* 11:142, 1962.

74. Mehendale, H.M. Modification of hepatobiliary function by toxic chemicals. *Fed. Proc.* 38:2240, 1979.

75. Anderson, J.W. and K. Ward Long-term effects of high-carbohydrate, high-fiber diets on glucose and lipid metabolism: A preliminary report on patients with diabetes. *Diabetes Care* 1:77, 1978.

76. McCarroll, A.M. and A.M. Connell. Effect of fiber on glucagon and gastrointestinal hormone responses in diabetics. *Program of the 39th Meeting of American Diabetes Association*, Los Angeles: 1979. Abstract 223.

77. Sims, E.A.H. and E.S. Horton. Endocrine and metabolic adaptation to obesity and starvation. *Am. J. Clin. Nutr.* 21:1455, 1968.

78. Sims, E.A.H., E. Danforth, Jr., E.S. Horton, G.A. Bray, J.A. Glennon and L.B. Salans. Endocrine and metabolic effects of experimental obesity in man. *Rec. Prog. Horm. Res.* 29:457, 1973.

79. Woods, S.C. and D. Porte, Jr. The central nervous system, pancreatic hormones, feeding and obesity. In *Advances in Metabolic Disorders*, edited by M. Miller and D.H. Bennett. New York: Academic Press, 1978, Vol. 9, p. 283.

80. Bagdade, J.D., E.L. Bierman and D. Porte, Jr. The significance of basal insulin levels in the evaluation of the insulin response to glucose in diabetic and nondiabetic subjects. *J. Clin. Invest.* 46:1549, 1967.

81. Stephan, F., P. Reville, P. Thierry and J.L. Schlienger Correlations between plasma insulin and body weight in obesity, anorexia nervosa and diabetes mellitus. *Diabetologia* 8:196, 1972.

82. Karam, J.H., G.M. Grodsky and P.H. Forsham. The relationship of obesity and growth hormone to serum insulin levels. *Ann. N.Y. Acad. Sci.* 131:374, 1965.

83. Grey, N. and D.M. Kipnis. Effect of diet composition on the hyperinsulinemia of obesity. *New Eng. J. Med.* 285:827, 1971.

84. Stern, J.S. and J. Hirsch. Obesity and pancreatic function. In *Handbook of Physiology, Endocrinology*, edited by D.F. Steiner. Washington: American Physiological Society, 1972, Vol. 1, p. 641.

85. Cahill, G.F. Diabetes and nutrition: Charaka Lecture in Diabetes. Edited by J.S. Bajaj. Amsterdam: Excerpta Medica, 1977, p. 32.

86. Nagulesparan, M., P. Savage and G.C. Johnson. Increased

in vivo insulin resistance to glucose disposal in glucose intolerant subjects is not due only to obesity. *Program of the 39th National Meeting of the American Diabetes Assn.* Los Angeles: 1979, p. 236.

87. Siiteri, P.K., J.E. Williams and N.K. Takaki. Steroid abnormalities in endometrial and breast carcinoma: a unifying hypothesis. *J. Steroid Bioch.* 87:897, 1976.

88. Barbato, A.L. and R.L. Landau. Testosterone deficiency of morbid obesity. *Clin. Res.* 22:647, 1974.

89. Amatruda, J.M., S.M. Harman, G. Pourmotabbed and D.H. Lockwood. Depressed plasma testosterone and fractional binding of testosterone in obese males. *J. Clin. Endocrinol. Metab.* 47:268, 1978.

90. Glass, A.R., R.S. Swerdioff, G.A. Bray, W.T. Dahms and R.L. Atkinson. Low serum testosterone and sex-hormone-binding-globulin in massively obese men. *J. Clin. Endocrinol. Metab.* 45:1211, 1977.

91. Schneider, G., M.A. Kirschner, R. Berknowitz and N.H. Ertel. Increased estrogen production in obese men. *J. Clin. Endocrinol. Metab.* 48:633, 1979.

92. Kley, H.K., H.G. Solback, J.C. McKinnan and H.L. Kruskember. Testosterone decrease and estrogen increase in male patients with obesity. *Acta Endocrinol.* 91:553, 1979.

93. Stanik, S., S.G. Korenman, L. Dornfeld and M.H. Maxwell. Weight loss normalizes the sex steroid imbalance of obese men. *Program of the 60th Annual Meeting of the Endocrine Society.* Miami, Florida: 1978, p. 204.

94. Crowther, J.S., B.S. Drasar, P. Goddard, M.J. Hill and K. Johnson. The effect of a chemically defined diet on the fecal flora and fecal steroid concentration. *Gut* 14:790, 1973.

95. Goddard, P. and M.J. Hill. The in vivo metabolism of cholesterol by gut bacteria in rat and guinea pig. *J. Steroid Biochem.* 5:569, 1974.

96. Lombardi, P., B. Goldin, E. Boutin and S.L. Gorback. Metabolism of androgens and estrogens by human fecal micro-organisms. *J. Steroid Biochem.* 9:795, 1978.

97. Taylor, W. The excretion of steroid metabolites in bile and feces. *Vit. Horm.* 29:201, 1971.

98. Latikainen, I. Review of Literature Biliary excretion and enterohepatic circulation of oestrogens. *Ann. Clin. Res. 2* (supplement): 7, 1970.

99. Gherman, M., G. Schneider, J. Winter and M.A. Kirschner. Acute effects of weight loss on sex hormone binding globulin levels in obese men. Abstract in the *Program of the Sixth International Congress of Endocrinology.* Melbourne, Australia: 1980.

100. Longcope, C. Metabolic clearance and blood production rates of estrogens in postmenopausal women. *Am. J. Obstet. Gynecol.* 111:778, 1971.

101. Nimrod, A. and K.J. Ryan. Aromatization of androgen by human abdominal and breast fat tissue. *J. Clin. Endocrinol. Metab.* 40:367, 1975.

102. Edman, C.C., E.J. Aiman, J.C. Porter and P.C. Macdonald The identification of estrogen product of extraglandular aromatization of plasma androstenedione. *Am J. Obstet. Gynecol.* 130:439, 1978.

103. Macdonald, P.C., C.D. Edman, D.L. Hemsell, J.G. Porter and P.K. Siiteri. Effect of obesity on conversion of plasma androstenedione to estrone in post-menopausal women with and without endometrial cancer. *Am. J. Obstet. Gynecol.* 130:448, 1978.

104. Pria, S.D., P.E. Lebech, D.C. McEwin, F.P. Rhoades, M. Furuhjelm, I. Bernard and P.G. McDonough. Hormone therapy of the menopause: A panel. In *The Menopausal Syndrome*, edited by R.B. Greenblatt, V.B. Mahesh, P.G. New York: Med. Com. Press, 1974, p. 197.

105. Edman, C.D., P.C. Macdonald. Effect of obesity on conversion of plasma androstenedione to estrone in ovulatory and anovulatory young women. *Am. J. Obstet. Gynecol.* 130:456, 1978.

106. Takaki, N.K., P.K. Siiteri, J. Williams, D.R. Tredway, S.B. Lewis and T.A. Daane. The effect of weight loss on peripheral estrogen synthesis in obese men. *Intl. J. Obesity* 2:386, 1978.

107. *The Treatment of Diabetes Mellitus*, edited by E.P. Joslin, H.F. Root, P. White and A. Marble. Philadelphia: Lea Febiger, 1959.

108. Goldman, J.K., J.D. Schnatz, L.L. Bernadis and L.A. Frohman. Effect of ventromedial hypothalamic destruction in rats with pre-existing streptozotocin-induced diabetes. *Metabolism* 21:132, 1972.

109. Powley, T.L. and C.A. Opsahl. Ventromedial hypothalamic obesity abolished by subdiaphragmatic vagotomy. *Am. J. Physiol.* 226:25, 1974.

110. Opsahl, C.A. and T.L. Powley. Failure of vagotomy to reverse obesity in the genetically obese Zucker rat. *Am. J. Physiol.* 226:34, 1974.

111. Tuohimaa, P. and M. Niemi. In vivo uptake of tritiated sex steroids by the hypothalamus of adult male rats treated neonatally with an antiandrogen (cyproterone). *Acta Endocrinol.* 71:45, 1974.

112. Okato, J. and C.A. Villee. Preferential uptake of estradiol by the anterior hypothalamus of the rat. *Endocrinol.* 80:567, 1967.

113. Tuohima, P. and R. Johansson. Decreased estradiol bind-

ing in the uterus and anterior hypothalamus of androgenized female rats. *Endocrinol.* 88:1159, 1971.

114. Kahwango, I., W.L. Heinrichs and W. Hermann. Isolation of oestradiol "receptors" from bovine hypothalamus and anterior pituitary gland. *Nature* 223:313, 1969.

115. Davis, P.G., B.S. McEwen and D.W. Pfaff. Localized behavioral effects of tritiated estradiol implants in the ventromedial hypothalamus of female rats. *Endocrinol.* 104:898, 1979.

116. Kato, J. Y, Atsum and M. Inaba. Development of estrogen receptors in the rat hypothalamus. *J. Biochem.* (Tokyo). 70:1051, 1971.

117. Baker, F.D. and C.L. Kragt. Maturation of the hypothalamic-pituitary-gonadal negative feedback system. *Endocrinol.* 85:522, 1969.

118. Leybold, K. and H.J. Staudinger. Sex difference in the steroid metabolism of rat liver cytoplasm. *Med Exp.* 2:46, 1960.

119. Gustafsson, J.A., M. Ingelman-Sundberg, A. Stenberg and F. Neumann. Partial feminization of hepatic steroid metabolism in male rats after neonatal administration of cyproterone acetate. *Biochem. J.* 64:267, 1975.

120. Gustafsson, J.A., M. Ingelman-Sundberg, A. Stenberg and T. Hokfelt. Feminization of hepatic steroid metabolism in male rats following electrothermic lesion of the hypothalamus. *Endocrinol.* 98:922, 1976.

121. Eriksson, H. Hormonal mechanisms regulating hepatic steroid metabolizing activities. Estrogenic induction of a corticosterone-metabolizing enzyme in the regenerating liver from castrated male rats. *Eur. J. Biochem.* 46:603, 1974.

122. Gustafsson, J.A., A. Mode, P. Skett and J. Hokfelt. Central control of a cytochrome P-450-dependant steroid hydroxylase in rat liver. In *Hormones and Brain Development*, edited by G. Dorner and K. Kawakami. Amsterdam:Elsevier–North Holland Biomedical Press, 1978, p. 129.

123. Fitzgerald, M.G., J.M. Malias, D.J. O'Sullivan and M. Wall. The effect of sex and parity on the incidence of diabetes mellitus. *Quart. J. Med.* 30:57, 1961.

124. Amendt, P., A. Mohnike and G. Dorner. On the significance of maternal diabetes in the pathogenesis of diabetes mellitus in offsprings. In *Hormones and Brain Development*, edited by G. Dorner and M. Kawakami. Amsterdam:Elsevier–North Holland, Biomedical Press, 1978, p. 305.

125. Dorner, G. and A. Mohnike. Zur bedeutur der perinatalen ubererahrung fur die pathogenese der Fettsucht und des diabetes mellitus. *Dt. Gesundh. Wesen.* 32:2325, 1977.

126. West, K.M. Detailed study of an epidemic of obesity and diabetes. *Program of American Diabetes Association 39th Annual Meeting.* Los Angeles: 1979, p. 385.

127. Schneider, G. Personal communication.

128. Ensenck, J.W. and R.H. Williams. Hormonal and nonhormonal factors modifying man's response to insulin. In *Handbook of Physiology, Endocrinology,* edited by D.F. Steiner. Washington: American Physiological Society, 1972, Vol. 1, p. 665.

129. Ciocirdia, C., M. Popa, I. Florea, A. Christoveanu, A. Tache, M. Bunia and S. Chirica. Adrenal and gonadal function in diabetic obese children with clinical features of moderate feminization. *Rev. Roum. Med. Endocrinol.* 17:49, 1979.

130. Jensen, S.B., C. Hagen, A. Froland and P.B. Pederson. Sexual function and pituitary axis in insulin treated diabetic men. *Acta Med. Scand. Suppl.* 624:65, 1979.

131. Charro-Salgado, A.L., B.F. Clark, C.H.L. Shackleton, L.J.P. Duncan and F.L. Mitchell. Urinary steroid excretory pattern in diabetes mellitus. *Lancet* i:126, 1968.

132. Goodner, C.J. and N. Freinkel. Studies of anterior pituitary tissue in vitro: effects of insulin and experimental diabetes mellitus upon carbohydrate metabolism. *J. Clin. Invest.* 40:261, 1961.

133. Dixit, P.K. and A. Lazarow. Effect of hyperglycemia and hypoglycemia on the glycogen content of the pituitary and adrenal glands of normal, subdiabetic and diabetic rats. *Endocrinol.* 71:745, 1962.

134. Distiller, L.A., J. Sagel, J.E. Morley, B.I. Joffe and H.C. Seftel. Pituitary responsiveness to luteinizing hormone-releasing hormone in insulin-dependent diabetes mellitus. *Diabetes* 24:378, 1975.

135. Savage, P.J., L.J. Bennion, E.V. Flock, M. Nagulesparan, D. Mott, J. Roth, R.H. Unger and P.H. Bennett. Diet-induced improvement of abnormalities in insulin and glucagon secretion and in insulin receptor binding in diabetes mellitus. *J. Clin. Endocrinol. Metab.* 48:999, 1979.

136. Trowell, H. Diabetes mellitus and dietary fiber of starchy foods. *Am J. Clin. Nutr.* 31:S53, 1978.

137. Trowell, H. The development of the concept of dietary fiber in human nutrition. *Am. J. Clin. Nutr.* 31:S3, 1978.

138. Jenkins, D.J.A., T.M.S. Wolever, T.D.R. Hockaday, A.R. Leeds, R. Howarth, S. Bacon, E.C. Apling and J. Dilawari. Treatment of diabetes with guar gum. Reduction in urinary glucose loss in diabetes. *Lancet* ii:779, 1977.

139. Trowell, H. Definition of dietary fiber and hypotheses that it is a protective factor in certain diseases. *Am. J. Clin. Nutr.* 29:417, 1976.

140. Roth, H.P. and M.A. Mehlman. Introduction. *Am. J. Clin. Nutr.* 31:S1, 1978.

141. Felig, P., J. Wahren and R. Hendler. Influence of oral glucose ingestion on splanchnic glucose and gluconeogenic substrate metabolism in man. *Diabetes* 24:568, 1975.

142. Felig, P. and J. Wahren. Influence of endogenous insulin secretion on splanchnic glucose and amino acid metabolism in man. *J. Clin. Invest.* 50:1702, 1971.

143. Wahren, J., P. Felig, E. Cesari and R. Luft. Splanchnic and peripheral glucose and amino acid metabolism in diabetes mellitus. *J. Clin. Invest.* 51:1870, 1972.

144. Felig, P., J. Wahren and R. Hendler. Influence of maturity-onset diabetes on splanchnic glucose balance after oral glucose ingestion. *Diabetes* 27:121, 1978.

145. Matschinsky, F.M., C.S. Hintz, K. Reichlmeier, B. Quistorff and B. Chance. The intralobular distribution of oxidized and reduced pyridine nucleotides in the liver of normal and diabetic rats. *Microenvirn. Metab. Compartments.* 5:149, 1978.

146. Adlercreutz, H. and R. Tenhunen. Some aspects of the interaction between natural and synthetic female sex hormones and the liver. *Am. J. Med.* 49:630, 1970.

147. Watanabe, H. Some factors in the biliary secretion of estrogens. *Adv. Steroid Biochem. Pharmacol.* 5:239, 1976.

148. Chopra, J.J., D. Tulchiasky and F.L. Greenway. Estrogen-androgen imbalance in hepatic cirrhosis. *Ann. Int. Med.* 79:198, 1973.

149. Baker, H.W.G., H.G. Burger, D.M. Dekretser, A. Dulmanis, B. Hudson, S. O'Connor, C.A. Paulson, N. Purcell, G.C. Rennie, C.S. Seah, H.P. Taft and C. Wang. A study of the endocrine manifestations of hepatic cirrhosis. *Quart. J. Med.* 45:145, 1976.

150. Kley, H.K., E. Nieschlag, W. Wiegelmann, H.G. Solbach and H.L. Kruskemper. Steroid hormones and their binding in plasma of male patients with fatty liver, chronic hepatitis and liver cirrhosis. *Acta Endocrinol.* 79:275, 1975.

151. Gordon, G.G., J. Olivo, F. Rafii and A.L. Southren. Conversion of androgens to estrogens in cirrhosis of the liver. *J. Clin. Endocrinol. Metab.* 40:1018, 1975.

152. Vanthiel, D.H., R. Lester and R. Sherins. Hypogonadism in alcoholic liver disease. Evidence for a double defect. *Gastroent.* 67:1188, 1974.

153. Gordon, G.G., K. Altman, A.L. Southren, E. Rubin and C.S. Lieber. Effect of alcohol on sex-hormone metabolism in normal men. *New Eng. J. Med.* 295:793, 1976.

154. Katzenellenbogen, B.S., T.S. Tsai, T. Tatee and J.A. Katz-

enellenbogen. Estrogen and antiestrogen action: studies in reproductive target tissues and tumors. In *Steroid Hormone Receptor Systems—Advances in Experimental Medicine and Biology*, edited by W.W. Leavitt, J.H. Clark. New York: Plenum Press, 1979, Vol. 117, p. 111.

155. Wittliff, J.L., P.H. Hedemann and W.M. Lewko. *Clinical Biochemistry of Cancer*. Washington: American Association of Clinical Chemistry, 1979, p. 179.

156. Cameron D., W. Stauffacher and A.E. Renold. Spontaneous hyperglycemia and obesity in laboratory rodents. In *Handbook of Physiology, Endocrinology*, edited by D.F. Steiner and N. Freinkel. Washington: American Physiological Society, 1972, Vol. 1, p. 611.

157. Samuels, L.T., R.M. Reinecke and H.A. Ball. Effect of diet on glucose tolerance and liver and muscle glycogen of hypophysectomized and normal rats. *Endocrinol.* 31:42, 1942.

158. Mickelson, O., S. Takahasi and C. Craig. Experimental obesity. I. Production of obesity in rats by feeding high-fat diets. *J. Nutr.* 57:541, 1955.

159. Nakhooda, A.F., A.A.A. Like, C.I. Chappell and E.B. Marliss. Metabolic and morphologic observations on the biobreeding spontaneously diabetic rat. *Clin. Res.* 23:638A, 1975.

160. Lemonnier, D, R. Aubert, J.P. Suquet and G. Rosselin. Metabolism of genetically obese rats on normal or high fat diet. *Diabetologia* 10:697, 1974.

161. Munger, B.L. and C.M. Lang. Spontaneous diabetes mellitus in guinea pigs. *Lab Invest.* 29:685, 1973.

162. Wolf, S. Diabetes mellitus animal model:Sekoke: Diabetes of nutritional origin in carp. *Am. J. Pathol.* 85:805, 1976.

163. Schmidt-Nielsen, K., H.B. Haines and D.B. Hackel. Diabetes mellitus in the sand rat induced by standard laboratory diets. *Science* 143:689, 1964.

164. Malaisse, W., F. Malaisse-Lagae, G.C. Gerritsen, W.E. Dulin and P.H. Wright. Insulin secretion in vitro by the pancreas of the Chinese hamster. *Diabetologia* 3:109, 1967.

165. Boquist, L. Obesity and pancreatic islet hyperplasia in the mongolian gerbil. *Diabetologia* 8:274, 1972.

166. Herberg, L. and D.L. Coleman. Laboratory animals exhibiting obesity and diabetes syndromes. *Metabolism* 26:59, 1977.

167. Stauffacher, W., L. Orci, D.P. Cameron, I.M. Burr and A.E. Renold. Spontaneous hyperglycemia and/or obesity in laboratory rodents: An example of the possible usefulness of animal disease models with both genetic and environmental components. *Rec. Progr. horm. Res.* 27:41, 1971.

168. Renold, A.E., D.P. Cameron, M. Amherdt, W. Stauffacher, E. Marliss, L. Orci and C. Rouiller. Endocrine-metabolic anomalies in rodents with hyperglycemic syndromes of hereditary and/or environmental origin. *Isr. J. Med. Sci.* 8:189, 1972.

169. Gerritsen, G.C., M.C. Blanks, R. Miller, and W.E. Dulin. Effect of diet limitation on the development of diabetes in prediabetic Chinese hamsters. *Diabetologia* 10:559, 1974.

170. Dulin, W.E. and G.C. Gerritsen. Interaction of genetics and environment on diabetes in the Chinese hamster as compared with human and other diabetic animal species. *Acta Diabetes Lat.* 9:supplement 1, 48, 1972.

171. Hellerstom, C., B. Hellman and S. Larsson. Some aspects of the structure and histochemistry of the adrenals in obese hyperglycemic mice. *Acta Pathol. Microbiol. Scand.* 54:365, 1962.

172. Kandutsch, A.A., D.L. Coleman and S.L. Alpert. Androgen effect on genetic and goldthioglucose-induced obesity. *Experientia* 28:473, 1972.

173. Wyse, B.M. and W.E. Dulin. The influence of age and dietary conditions on diabetes in the d b mouse. *Diabetologia* 6:268, 1970.

174. Iwatsaka, H., S. Taketomi, T. Matsuo and Z. Suzuoki. Congenitally impared hormone sensitivity of the adipose tissue of spontaneously diabetic mice KK validity of thrifty gentoype in KK mice. *Diabetologia* 10:611, 1974.

175. Howard, Jr., Ch. F. Diabetes in Macacanigra: metabolic and histologic changes. *Diabetologia* 10:671, 1974.

References

Chapter 2

Campbell, G.D. Connubial diabetes and the possible role of oral diabetogens. *Brit. Med. Journal* May 27, 1961, p. 538.

Cassidy, J.T. Diabetes in Fiji. *New Zealand Med. J.* 66:167, 1967.

Damon, A. Race, ethnic group, and disease. *Social Biol.* 16:69, 1969.

Hathorn, M., G. Gillman, G.D. Campbell. Blood lipides, mucoproteins and fibrinolytic activity in diabetic Indians and Africans in Natal. *Lancet* June 17, 1961, 1314.

Jackson, W.P.U. Epidemiology of diabetes in South Africa. In *Advances in Metabolic Disorders*, edited by M. Miller and P.H. Bennett. New York: Academic Press, 1978, Vol. 9, p. 112.

Kagan, A., B.R. Harris, W. Winkelstein Jr., K.G. Johnson, H. Kato, S.L. Syne, G.G. Rhoads, M.L. Gay, M.Z. Nickaman, H.B. Hamilton, and J.J. Tillotson. Comparison of Nutrient Intake of Japanese in Hawaii and Japanese in Japan. *Journal of Chronic Diseases*, 1974, Vol. 27, p. 345.

Kawate, R., M. Miyanishi, M. Yamakido, and Y. Nishimoto. Preliminary studies of the prevalence and mortality of diabetes mellitus in Japanese in Japan and on the island of Hawaii. In *Advances in Metabolic Disorders*, edited by M. Miller and P.H. Bennett. New York: Academic Press, 1978, Vol. 9, p. 201.

Kawate, R., M. Yamakido, Y. Nishimoto, P.H. Bennett, R.F. Hamman, and W.C. Knowler. Diabetes mellitus and its vascular complications in Japanese migrants on the island of Hawaii. *Diabetes Care* 2:161, 1979.

Medalie, J.H., J.B. Herman, V. Goldbourt, and C.M. Papier. Variations in incidence of diabetes among 10,000 adult Israeli males and the factors related to their development. In *Advances in Metabolic Disorders*, edited by M. Miller and P.H. Bennett. New York: Academic Press, 1978, Vol. 9, p. 94.

Poon-King, T., M.V. Henry, and F. Rampersad. Prevalence and natural history of diabetes in Trinidad. *Lancet* i:155, 1968.

Addanki, S. Roles of nutrition, obesity and estrogens in Diabetes Mellitus: Human leads to an experimental approach to prevention. *Preventive Medicine*, September 10, 1981.

Chapter 3

Diabetes Data, 1977, U.S. Dept. Health, Education, Welfare, Public Health Source, National Institutes of Health.

Health Interview Survey, 1964/65, 1965/66 and 1973. National Center for Health Statistics.

1971–72 Health and Nutrition Examination Survey, National Center for Health Statistics.

Malins, J.M., Pregnancy as a potent stress for diabetes. *Clin. Endocrine. Metabolism* 1:645–672 (1972).

Fitzgerald, M.G., J.M. Malins, D.J. O'Sullivan, and Mary Wall. The effect of sex and parity on the incidence of diabetes mellitus. *Quar. Journ. of Med.* New Series XXX, No. 117, Jan. 1961, pp. 57–70.

Rosenbloom, Charles, The natural history of diabetes mellitus. *Public Health Reviews* III: 2, 1973, pp. 131–132.

Edman, C.D., P.C. MacDonald. Effect of obesity on conversion of plasma androstenedione to estrone in ovulatory and anovulatory young women. *Am. J. Obstet. Gynecol.* 130:456 (1978).

Grodin, J.M., P.K. Siiteri, P.C. MacDonald. Source of estrogen production in postmenopausal women. *J. Clin. Endocrinol. Metab.* 36:207, 1973.

Nimrod, A. and K.J. Ryan. Aromatization of androgens by human abdominal and breast fat tissue. *J. Clin. Endocrinol. Metab.* 40:367, 1975.

MacDonald, P.C., C.D. Edman, D.L. Hemsell, J.C. Porter, and P.K. Siiteri. Effect of obesity on conversion of plasma androstenedione to estrone in postmenopausal women with and without endometrial cancer. *Am. J. Obstet. Gynecol.* 130:448, 1978.

Spellacy, W.N., W.C. Buhi, and S.A. Birk. The effect of estrogens on carbohydrate metabolism: glucose, insulin, and growth hormone studies on one hundred and seventy-one women ingesting premarin, mestranol and ethinyl estradiol for six months. *Am. J. Obstet. Gynecol.* 114: 3, 1972, p. 378.

Edman, C.D., E.J. Aiman, J.C. Porter, and P.C. MacDonald. Identification of the estrogen product of extraglandular aromatization of plasma androstenedione. *Am. J. Obstet. Gynecol.* 130:439, 1978.

Schindler, A.E., A. Ebert, and E. Friedrich. Conversion of androstenedione to estrone by human breast fat tissue. *J. Clin. Endocrinol Metab.* 35:627, 1972.

Longscope, C. Metabolic clearance and blood production rates of estrogens in postmenopausal women. *Am. J. Obstet. Gynecol.* 111:778, 1971.

Takaki, N.K., P.K. Siiteri, J. Williams, D.R. Tredway, S.B. Lewis, and T.A. Daane. The effect of weight loss on peripheral estrogen synthesis in obese women. *International J. Obesity* 2:386, 1978.

Goldin, Barry R., Herman Adlercreutz, Johanna T. Dwyer, Linda Swenson, James H. Warram, and Sherwood L. Gorbach. The effect of diet on excretion of estrogens in pre and postmenopausal women. Paper presented during fat and cancer workshop in Bethesda, Maryland, 1979.

Wyeth Laboratories, Inc. Detailed patient labeling "What you should know about oral contraceptives," C1 2981–2, 9/25/78.

Ostrander, Leon D., Jr., Donald E. Lamphiear, Walter D. Block, George W. Williams, and Wendy J. Carmen. Oral contraceptives and physiological variables. *J.A.M.A.* 244: 677:679, 1980.

Spellacy, William N. A review of carbohydrate metabolism and the oral contraceptives. *Am. J. Obstet. Gynecol.* 104: 3, 1969, p. 448.

Yen, S.S.C., and P. Vela. Effects of contraceptive steroids on carbohydrate metabolism. *J. Clin. Endocrin.* 28:1564, 1968.

Chapter 4

Teplitz, Jerry, "Managing your stress", cassette program 214, 78th Street, Virginia Beach, VA.

Wicking, J., M. Ringrose, S. Whitehouse, and P. Zimmet. The Funafuti Study. *Diabetes Care* 4:92, 1981.

Cheraskin, E. and W.M. Ringsdorf, Jr. *Psychodietetics.* New York: Bantam, 1976.

Reuben, David. *Everything You Always Wanted to Know about Nutrition.* New York: Avon, 1977.

Chapter 5

Van Itallie, Theodore B. Dietary fiber and obesity. *Am. J. Clin, Nutrit.* 31:9, 1978, pp. S45–S52.

Albrink, Margaret J. Cultural and endocrine origins of obesity. *Am. J. Clin. Nutr.* 21: 12, 1968, pp. 1398–1403.

Sims, Ethan A.H., Ralph F. Goldman, Charles M. Gluck, Edward S. Horton, Phillip C. Kelleher, and David W. Rowe. Experimental obesity in man. *Transactions of the Assoc. of Am. Physicians,* Session 81, 1968.

Woods, Stephen C., et al. Metabolic hormones and regulation of body weight. Psychology Reviews, 81, 1974, p. 26.

Karam, John H., Gerald M. Grodsky, Peter H. Forsham. Insulin Secretion in Obesity: Pseudodiabetes? *Am. J. Clin. Nutrit.* 21:12, 1968, 1445–1454.

Woods, Stephen C., and Daniel Porte, Jr. Neural contact of endocrine pancreas. *Psychological Reviews* 54:3, 1974.

Carpenter, Paul. Man's "Sex drive not all downhill after 70." AP, *Columbus* Dispatch A–5, Mar. 22, 1981.

Bagdade, J.D., E.L. Bierman, and D. Porte. Correlation between urinary estradiol production and basal immunoreactive insulin in obese men. *J. Clin. Invest.* 46:1549, 1967.

Chapter 7

Bancroft, John and F.C.W. Wu. Diabetic Impotence. *British Medical Journal*, February 16, 1980, p. 483.

Deutsch, Stanley and Lawrence Sherman. Previously Unrecognized Diabetes Mellitus in Sexually Impotent Men. *J.A.M.A.* 244:21, 1980.

Hosking, B., E. Hampton, R. Clark, and S. Robertson. Diabetic Impotence: Studies of Nocturnal Erection during REM Sleep. *British Medical Journal*, December 1, 1979.

Kolodny, R.C., C.E. Kahn, and H.H. Goldstein. Sexual Dysfunction in Diabetic Men. *Diabetes* 23, 1974, pp. 306–309.

Sacerdote, Alan and, Sheldon J. Bleicher. Sexual Dysfunction in Diabetes Mellitus. Personal communication.

Schiavi, Raul C. Psychological Treatment of Erectile Disorders in Diabetic Patients. *Annals of Internal Medicine* 92 (Part 2), 1980.

Chapter 8

Harwood, R. Severe diabetes with remission—report of a case and review of the literature. *New Engl. J. Med.* 257: 257–261, 1957.

Genuth, Saul M. Clinical remission in diabetes mellitus, studies of insulin secretion. *Diabetes* 19:2, 1970.

Mann, J.I. Diet and diabetes. *Diabetologia* 18:89–95, 1980.

Singh, Inder. Low fat diet and therapeutic doses of insulin in diabetes mellitus. *Lancet*, Feb. 26, 1955.

Anderson, James W., Susan K. Ferguson, Dennis Karounos, Linda O'Malley, Beverly Sieling, and Wen-ju Lin Chen. Mineral and vitamin status on high-fiber diets: Long-term studies of diabetic patients. *Diabetes Care* 3:1, 1980, pp. 38.

Anderson, James W. and Kyleen Ward. High-carbohydrate, high-fiber diets for insulin-treated men with diabetes mellitus. *Am. J. Clin. Nutr.* 32, 1979, pp. 2312–2321.

Anderson, James W., Wendy R. Midgley, and Betty Wedman. Fiber and diabetes. *Diabetes Care* 2:4, 1979.

Anderson, James W. High fiber diets offer promise for persons with diabetes. Public forum, University of Toronto, May 17, 1979.

Anderson, James W. and Kyleen Ward. Long term effects of high-carbohydrate, high-fiber diets on glucose and lipid metabolism: A preliminary report on patients with diabetes. *Diabetes Care* 1:2, 1978.

Kiehm, Tae G., James W. Anderson, and Kyleen Ward. Beneficial effects of a high-carbohydrate, high-fiber diet on hyperglycemic diabetic men *Am. J. Clin. Nutr.* 29, 1976, pp. 895–899.

Anderson, James W., Wen-ju Lin Chen, and Beverly Sieling. Hypolipidemic effects of high-carbohydrate, high-fiber diets *Metabolism* 29:6, 1980.

Anderson, James W. and Wen-ju Lin Chen. Plant fiber. Carbohydrate and lipid metabolism. *Am. J. Clin. Nutr.* 32, 1979, pp. 346–363.

Trowell, Hugh. Diabetes mellitus and dietary fiber of starchy foods. *Am. J. Clin. Nutr.* 31:S53–S57, 1978.

Brunzell, John D., Roger L. Lerner, William R. Hazzard, Daniel Porte, and Edwin L. Bierman. Improved glucose tolerance with high-carbohydrate feeding in mild diabetes. *New Engl. Journ. Med.* 284:10, 1971.

Jenkins, David J.A., T.D.R. Hockaday, Richard Howarth, et al. Treatment of diabetes with guar gum. *Lancet,* Oct. 15, 1977.

Simpson, H.C.R., S. Lousley, and M. Geekie. A high carbohydrate leguminous fibre diet improves all aspects of diabetic control. *Lancet,* Jan. 3, 1981.

Miranda, Perla M. and David L. Horwitz. High fiber diets in the treatment of diabetes mellitus. *Annals of Intern. Med.* 88:482–486, 1978.

Monnier, L., T.C. Pham, L. Aquirre, et al. Influences of indigestible fibers on glucose tolerance. *Diabetes Care,* 1:83–88, 1978.

Goulder, T.J. and K.G.M.M. Alberti. Dietary fiber and diabetes. *Diabetologia* 15:285–287, 1978.

Antonis, A. and I. Bersohn. The influence of diet on serum triglycerides. *Lancet,* Jan. 7, 1961.

Groen, J.J., K.B. Tijong, M. Koster, et al. The influence of nutrition and ways of life on blood cholesterol and the prevalence of hypertension and coronary heart disease among Trappist and Benedictine Monks. *Am. J. Clin. Nutr.* 10: 1962.

Shaper, A.G. and K.W. Jones. Serum cholesterol, diet, and coronary heart disease in Africans and Asians in Uganda. *Lancet,* Oct. 10, 1959.

Gherman, M., G. Schneider, J. Winter, et al. Acute effects of weight loss on sex hormone binding globulin levels in obese men. Abstract: Sixth International Congress of Endocrinology, 1980.

Hemmes, Richard B., Susan Hubsch, and Howard M. Pack.

High dosage of testosterone propionate increases litter production of the genetically obese male Zucker rat. *Proceedings of the Soc. for Exper. Biol. and Med.* 159:424–427, 1978.

O'Dea, John P.K., Ralph G. Wieland, Marvin C. Hallberg, et al. Effect of dietary weight loss on sex steroid binding, sex steroids, and gonadotropins in obese postmenopausal women. *J. Lab. Clin. Med.* 93:1004, 1979.

Chapter 9

Long, Ruth Yale. *Nutrition and Cancer.* Nutrition Education Association, Inc., 1979.

Long, Ruth Yale. *No More Cancer,* second ed. Nutrition Education Assoc., Inc., 1979.

Long, Ruth Yale. *Nutrition and Cancer Update.* Nutrition Education Assoc., Inc., 1980.

Fredricks, Carlton. *Breast Cancer: A Nutritional Approach,* New York: Grosset and Dunlap, 1977.

Wellman, Klaus F. and Bruno W. Volk. *The Diabetic Pancreas* (chap: Cancer and Diabetes) New York: Plenum Press, 1977.

Reddy, Bandaru S., Leonard A. Cohen, David G. McCoy, Peter Hill, John H. Weisburger, and Ernst L. Wynder. *Nutrition and Its Relationship to Cancer, Advances in Cancer Research.* Vol. 32 New York: Academic Press, Inc., 1980.

Armstrong, B. and R. Doll. *Int. J. Cancer,* 15:617–631, 1975.

Cole, P., D. Cramer, S. Yen, MacMahon B. Paffenbarger, and J. Brown. Environmental Factors and Cancer Incidence and Mortality in Different Countries and Special Reference to Dietary Practices. *Cancer Res.* 38:745–748, 1978.

Volk, Bruno W. and Klaus F. Wellman. *Cancer and Diabetes, the Diabetic Pancreas.* New York: Plenum Press, 1977.

Miller, Anthony B. An overview of hormone associated cancers. *Cancer Research* 38:3985–3990, 1978.

Nomura, Abraham, Brian E. Henderson, and James Lee. Breast cancer and diet among the Japanese in Hawaii. *Am. J. Clin. Nutr.* 31:2020–2025, 1978.

Chapter 10

Joslin, E.P., H.F. Root, P. White, and A. Marble. "*The Treatment of Diabetes Mellitus.*" Philadelphia: Lea and Fediger, 1959.

Podolsky, Stephen and M. Viswanathan. *Secondary Diabetes: The Spectrum of the Diabetic Syndromes.* New York Raven Press, 1980.

Duncan, Theodore, G. *The Good Life with Diabetes,* Philadelphia: Duncan Foundation, 1973.

Cheraskin, E. and W.M. Ringsdorf, Jr. *Psychodietetics*. New York: Bantam 1974.

Pritikin, N. *The Pritikin Program for Diet and Exercise*. New York: Bantam, 1979.

Chapter 11

Pritikin, N. *The Pritikin Program for Diet and Exercise*. New York: Bantam, 1979.

Cheraskin, E. and W.M. Ringsdorf, Jr. *Psychodietetics*. New York: Bantam, 1974.

Van Thiel, David H., Judith S. Gavaler, Roger Lester, D. Lynn Loriaux, and Glenn D. Braunstein. Plasma estrone, prolactin, neurophysin, and sex steroid-binding globulin in chronic alcoholic men. *Metabolism* 24:9, 1975.

Kley, H.K., E. Nieschlag, W. Wiegelmann, H.G. Solbach, and H.L. Krüskemper. Steroid hormones and their binding in plasma of male patients with fatty liver, chronic hepatitis, and liver cirrhosis. *Acta Endocrinologica*, 79, 1975, 275–285.

Gordon, Gary G., Jaime Olivo, Rafii Fereidoon, and A. Louis Southren. Conversion of androgens to estrogens in cirrhosis of the liver. *J. Clin. Endocrinol. Metab.* 40:1018, 1975.

Chopra, Inder J., Dan Tulchinsky, and Frank L. Greenway. Estrogen-androgen imbalance in hepatic cirrhosis. *Annals of Internal Medicine* 79:198–203, 1973.

Gordon, Gary G., Kurt Altman, Louis A. Southren, Emanuel Rubin, and Charles S. Lieber. Effect of alcohol (ethanol) administration on sex hormone metabolism in normal men. *N. Engl. J. Med.* 295:793–797, 1976.

Chapter 12

Lindner, Peter G. As seen by a doctor. *Obesity and Bariatric Medicine*. 3:4, 1974.

To the Newcomer. Overeaters Anonymous, Inc., 1979.

To the Family of the Compulsive Overeater. O.A., Inc., 1979.

Good Nutrition: A vital Ingredient of Abstinence. O.A., Inc., 1979.

Moving toward Recovery with the Dignity of Choice. O.A., Inc., 1979.

Before You Take That First Compulsive Bite Remember . . . O.A. Inc., 1973.

Welcome Back. O.A., Inc., 1979.

A program of Recovery. O. A., Inc., 1979.

A Commitment to Abstinence. O.A., Inc., 1973.

Abstinence Guide for Maintainers. O.A., Inc., 1976.

Chapter 13

National Dairy Council Digest, Nutrition and Vegetarianism. 50:1, 1979.

Dwyer, Johanna T., Laura Mayer, D.V.H., Randy Francis Kandel, and Jean Mayer. The new vegetarians. *J. Am. Dietetic. Assoc.* 62, May, 1973.

Dwyer, Johanna T., Laura Mayer, D.V.H., Kathryn Dowd, Randy F. Kandel, and Jean Mayer. The new vegetarians: The natural high? *Research* 65, Nov., 1974.

Dwyer, Johanna T., Ruth Palombo, Halorie Thorne, Isabelle Valadian, and Robert B. Reed. Preschoolers on alternate life-style diets. *Research, J. Am. Dietetic. Assoc.* 72, Mar. 1978.

Dwyer, Johanna T. Randy F. Kandel, Laura Mayer, D.V.H., and Jean Mayer. The "new" vegetarians. *Research, J. Am. Dietetic Assoc.* 64, 1974.

Register, U.D., and L.M. Sonnenberg. The vegetarian diet. *J.Am. Dietetic Assoc.* 62:1973.

Vegetarian diet and vitamin B_{12} deficiency. *Nutrition Reviews.* 36:8, 1978.

Todhunter, Neige E. "Food habits, food faddism and nutrition." In *Food Nutrition and Health. World Review of Nutrition and Dietetics,* ed. by M. Rechcigl Vol. 16:pp. 286–317. Washington: Karger, Basel, 1973.

Ruys, J. and J.B. Hickie. Serum cholesterol and triglyceride levels in Australian adolescent vegetarians. *Short Reports. British Med. Journ.* 10, July 1976, pp. 87.

West, Raymond O., and Olive B. Hayes. Diet and serum cholesterol levels. *Am. J. Clin. Nutrit.* 21:8, 1968, pp. 853–862.

Phillips, Roland L., Frank R. Lemon, Lawrence W. Beeson, and Jan W. Kuzma. Coronary heart disease mortality among Seventh-day Adventists with differing dietary habits: a preliminary report. *Am. J. Clin. Nutrit.* 31, Oct. 1978, pp. S191–198.

Sanders, T.A.B., Frey R. Ellis, and J.W.T. Dickerson. Studies of Vegans: the fatty acid composition of plasma choline phosphoglycerides, erythrocytes, adipose tissue, and breast milk and some indicators of susceptibility to ischemic heart disease in vegans and omnivore controls. *Am. J. Clin. Nutr.* 31:805–813.

Vyhmeister, Irma B., U.D. Register, and Lydia M. Sonnenberg. Safe vegetarian diets for children. *Ped. Clinics of N. Amer.* 24:1, 1977.

Committee on Nutrition. Nutritional aspects of vegetarianism, Health foods, and fad diets. *Pediatrics,* 59:3, 1977.

Harland, Barbara F. and Michael Peterson. Nutritional status of lacto-ovo-vegetarian Trappist Monks. *Research,* 72, March 1978.

Chapter 14

Benowicz, Robert J. *Vitamins and You*. New York: Grosset & Dunlap, 1979.

Di Cyan, Erwin. *Vitamins in Your Life*. New York: Simon & Schuster, 1974.

Nutrition Search, Inc. *Nutrition Almanac*. New York: McGraw-Hill, 1979.

Marks, John, M.D. *A Guide to the Vitamins—Their Role in Health and Disease*. Lancaster, England: Medical & Technical Publishing, 1978.

Glossary

ACIDOSIS—Decreased alkalinity of the blood and tissues

AEROBIC—Living, active, or present in oxygen

AMINO ACIDS—The building blocks of proteins

ANAEROBIC—Not needing oxygen for life

ANDROGENS—Male hormones

AROMATIZATION—A chemical conversion characterized by the forming of a double bond

ARTERIOSCLEROSIS—A chronic thickening and hardening of the arterial walls

ATHEROSCLEROSIS—Degenerative disease of the arteries, a stage of arteriosclerosis

AUTOPSY—A postmortem examination

BASAL METABOLISM—The amount of energy used in a fasting and resting organism to maintain respiration, circulation, and cellular activity

BEHAVIOR MODIFICATION—Permanent changes in a life-style

BIOFEEDBACK—Seeing or hearing signals representing various body functions in order to learn to control these functions

BILE—A digestive fluid secreted by the liver

BIOPSY—Removal of tissue from a living body for examination

BLOOD-SUGAR LEVEL—The number of milligrams of glucose in each deciliter of blood.

BULIMIA—Abnormal hunger and craving for food

CAFFEINE—A stimulant, found in coffee, tea, and colas, which acts on the central nervous system

CALORIE—A measure of the energy contained in food

CAPILLARIES—The small blood vessels that connect arteries and veins and nourish the cells

CARBOHYDRATES—Chemicals composed of carbon, oxygen, and hydrogen, such as starches, sugars, and some fibers

CARCINOGEN—A substance that causes cancer

CELLULOSE—A carboyhdrate fiber found in plants

CHEMOTHERAPY—The treatment of disease (especially cancer) with chemicals

CHOLESTEROL—A fat-soluble alcohol which is an essential part of body cells and fluids

COLON—The large bowel connecting the small intestine to the anus

CORONARY—Relating to the arteries that supply blood to the heart

CUSHING'S DISEASE—A disease of pituitary or adrenal glands and characterized by obesity of the head, neck, and trunk

DIABETES MELLITUS—A disorder characterized by hyperglycemia, glycosuria, polyuria, thirst, and weight loss

DIET SABOTAGE—The frustrating, for selfish reasons, of another's attempts to follow a dietary regimen

DIURETIC—Tending to increase the flow of urine

DIVERTICULOSIS—A disorder characterized by abnormal blind sacs or pouches in the intestine wall

ENDOCRINE—Relating to ductless glands that secrete into the bloodstream

ENDOGENOUS—Originating within the body

ENDOMETRIAL—Relating to the mucous-membrane lining of the uterus

ESTRADIOL—A female hormone produced in the placenta during pregnancy

ESTROGENS—Female hormones

ESTRONE—A female hormone produced in obese tissues, the ovaries, and the adrenal glands

EXCRETION—The elimination of useless or harmful matter from the body

EXOGENOUS—Originating outside the body

FAST—A period of no ingestion of food; to abstain from food

FAT—Glycerides of fatty acids, soluble in ether, found in adipose tissue of animals and oil seeds

FECES—Bodily waste discharged through the anus

FETUS—A developing but unborn vertebrate; an unborn human from three months after conception to birth

FIBER—The undigestible or semidigestible part of plant foods

FLATULENCE—Gas in the digestive tract

FLORA—Bacteria inhabiting the digestive tract of humans

FROHLICH'S SYNDROME OR DISEASE—Adiposogenital dystrophy, a neuromuscular disorder of the genitals

GASTRIC STAPLING—A drastic weight-loss treatment involving permanent altering of the digestive tract

GENETIC—Passed from parent to child through chemical information within the egg and sperm

GLUCOSE—A sugar in the blood that provides energy to the tissues

GLUCOSE INTOLERANCE—Abnormal reaction of the metabolism to a meal of sugar (glucose)

GLUCOSE TOLERANCE TEST—Giving a sugar (glucose) meal and then measuring the blood glucose level for several hours

GLYCOGEN—The principal form in which carbohydrate is stored in animal tissues

GONAD—A primary sex gland; testes or ovaries

HEART ATTACK—The death of part of the tissue of the heart

HEMICELLULOSE—A type of plant fiber or polysaccharide

HIGH DENSITY LIPOPROTEIN (HDL)—A combination of fat and protein, with more protein than fat

HORMONE—An organic product of living cells which travels to other parts of the organism and causes specific cellular effects to occur

HYDROLYZATION—A chemical decomposition in which elements of water split the molecules of another substance and combine with the parts of that second substance

HYPER—Too much or too many

HYPERGLYCEMIA—Too much glucose in the blood

HYPERINSULINEMIA—An excess of insulin in the bloodstream

HYPERLIPEMIA—Too many fatty substances in the blood

HYPERPHAGIA—Abnormally increased desire for food—usually cause by lesion to the hypothalamus

HYPERPLASIA—Abnormal cell multiplication and growth

HYPERTENSION—High blood pressure

HYPERTRIGLYCERIDEMIA—Too many triglycerides (fats containing 3 fatty acids) in the blood

HYPO—Too little or not enough

HYPOGLYCEMIA—Too little glucose in the blood

HYPOTHALAMUS—Part of the brain which controls hunger, satiety, and stress

IMPOTENCE—A male's inability to perform the sex act

INCIDENCE—The number of new cases of a disease for a given population and time period

INSULIN—A protein hormone secreted by the pancreas, needed for carbohydrate metabolism

INSULIN RESISTANCE—The refusal of the cells to accept glucose because of the presence of antagonizing factors such as estrogens circulating in the bloodstream

INTESTINAL BYPASS—A drastic surgical weight-loss treatment wherein a section of intestine is removed

INTESTINAL MICROFLORA—Small bacteria in the digestive tract

ISCHEMIC—Lacking a supply of blood to the heart

IRRADIATION—Treatment (especially of cancer) by exposure to X-rays, radium rays, or other radiation

IN VITRO—Outside a living body

IN VIVO—In the living body of an animal or plant

JUVENILE ONSET—Diabetes mellitus occurring between the ages of two and four and usually requiring insulin administration

KETOACIDOSIS—Ketones and acids in high concentration in the body

KETONES—Chemical products of fat digestion containing a carbonyl group, CO

KETOSIS—Too high a concentration of ketones in the tissues and fluids of the body

LESION—An abnormal structural change in a body part due to injury or disease

LIBIDO—Sexual drive, interest, or urge

LIGNIN—A fiber, part of the woody cell walls of plants

LIPIDS—Same as **FAT**

LIVER—A large organ which secretes bile and makes various changes on blood contents

LOW BLOOD SUGAR—Less than 80 mg. of glucose per 100 ml. of blood

LOW DENSITY LIPOPROTEIN (LDL)—A combination of fat and protein, with relatively more fat

LOW-FAT—Containing as little fat as possible or necessary; in a diet, under 15 percent

LUMEN—The opening or cavity of a tubular organ such as the intestine

MALIGNANT—Cancerous

MATURITY ONSET—Diabetes mellitus starting at age twenty-four and up

MENARCHE—The onset of menstruation or puberty in the female

MENOPAUSE—When menstruation and the reproductive ability ceases in the female

METABOLISM—The sum of the process by which a particular substance is handled in the living organism

NEUROPATHY—Abnormal degenerative states of the nervous system

NICOTINE—A poisonous liquid alkaloid found in tobacco

NON-FAT—Containing no fat

OBESE—Weighing more than 20 percent over your ideal body weight, based on the Metropolitan life Assurance tables

OSTEOPOROSIS—A nutritional disorder characterized by a decrease in bone mass and resulting fragility

OVEREATERS ANONYMOUS—A mutual support group for compulsive overeaters

PANCREAS—The gland that produces insulin, glucagon, and digestive enzymes

PATHOLOGY—The study of abnormality and disease

PECTIN—A plant fiber

PERIPHERAL—Located at or near the surface of the body

PERISTALSIS—Waves of involuntary contractions of the intestine, which move the contents

PITUITARY—An endocrine organ which secretes substances that control other endocrine organs, growth and development, smooth muscle and liver function, reproductive organs, and most basic body functions

PLACENTA—The vascular organ that permits the exchange of substances between maternal and fetal blood

POLYSACCHARIDES—Complex carbohydrates

POLYUNSATURATED—Not saturated with hydrogen; usually such fats are liquid at room temperature

PRESERVATIVE—A substance added to foods to protect them from decay or spoilage

PREVALENCE—Number of known cases of a disease affecting a certain population

PROGESTERONE—A female hormone found in the corpus luteum

PROLACTIN—The hormone needed to make natural mother's milk

PROSTATE—A gland surrounding the male urethra

PROTEIN—Complex combinations of amino acids that are the essential constituents of living cells

REMISSION—The complete disappearance of a disease or disorder

RECEPTOR—A special area on a cell which receives signals from the contents of the blood

REFINED CARBOHYDRATE—A carbohydrate food from which the minerals, vitamins, and fiber have been taken through processing

SATURATED FAT—Fat fully combined with hydrogen, usually solid at room temperature

SERUM CHOLESTEROL—The level of cholesterol in the blood

SERUM TRIGLYCERIDE—The level of triglycerides in the blood

SIMPLE CARBOHYDRATE—Mono- and di-saccharides; sugar

SHBG (SSBG)—Sex-hormone-(steroid)-binding globulin, binds with and deactivates steroids in the blood

STEROID—Hormone

STOOL—Feces, human solid waste products from the colon

STRESS—A physical, chemical, or emotional factor that causes physical tension and often disease

STROKE—Hemorrhage in a blood vessel in (or supplying) the brain, and the resulting damage

TESTOSTERONE—Male hormone

THYROID—An endocrine gland that helps control growth and metabolism

TOXIC—Poisonous

TRANQUILIZER—A drug that calms emotionally without affecting thought processes

TRIGLYCERIDE—A combination of three fatty acids

UNSATURATED FATTY ACID—Fats or oils not saturated with hydrogen, usually liquid at room temperature

UREA—A product of protein metabolism found in urine

URETHRA—The canal that carries the urine from the bladder to the outside of the body

VITAMIN—Organic compounds found in food, which are necessary for body metabolism

VAGUS (NERVE)—The tenth cranial nerve supplying the viscera (including the pancreas).

Index

226

HELP YOURSELF
To Bestsellers from Pinnacle